SWEET & SOUR: A DIABETIC LIFE

SWEET & SOUR: A DIABETIC LIFE

Peter Corris

ISBN-13: 9781517510695

*For giving of their knowledge and providing
information from my medical records, thanks to Drs
Paul Beaumont, John Burgess, Warren Kidson and
Gordon Ennis. Thanks also to Ruth Corris.*

In memory of Fred Hollows

CONTENTS

PHOTOGRAPHS

1. 1958, aged 16, shortly after I was diagnosed with diabetes.
2. 1968, looking plump in Canberra.
3. Roughing it at Wanderer Bay, Guadalcanal, Solomon Islands, 1969.
4. Passport photo, 1970 – this look plus needles and syringe aroused suspicion at Moscow airport.
5. Boozy in Canberra, 1973.
6. After a lasering session, 1977, in Sydney with my four-month-old daughter, Ruth.
7. After a dressing down from Fred Hollows, running with four-minute-miler Merv Lincoln, 1980. (Courtesy Fairfax Photo Library.)
8. 1998, 40 years a diabetic – fit and well with Jean on Coochiemudlo Island, Queensland.
   (Courtesy Queensland Newspapers Pty Ltd.)

Cover Photograph - Peter Corris' plaque at the Sydney Writers' Walk, Circular Quay, Sydney

INTRODUCTION

This is not a 'how to live with diabetes' book. It contains no recipes, no diets, no advice about injection equipment or technique. Excellent books on the management of diabetes are available in any good library[1] and many public hospitals now have first-rate diabetic support services. On the Internet my usual search engine throws up 14 categories and 409 sites for 'diabetes'. A telephone call to Diabetes Australia can supply the diabetic or his or her carers with all the information needed to allow the diabetic to lead a close to normal life.

And yet all this support and information can be seen as somewhat clinical, and I'm encouraged to think that an intimate, frank account of one person's experience as a diabetic might serve some purpose.

At the time of writing I've been a diabetic for 41 years. Broadly speaking, I spent the first half of this time behaving precisely as a diabetic should not, and set myself on a course that would have led to blindness, amputation and an early death. I have spent the second half behaving as a diabetic should. This journey has provided the structure for this book a long downward swoop and an upturn just in time.

The approach is basically biographical: I've sketched the events of my life and tried to outline the part diabetes has played in shaping those events for better or worse. When I look back I see how foolish I was to neglect my diabetes as I did and how lucky I've been to escape the worst consequences of that neglect. As I examine my life now I realise that being a 'good diabetic' is not so difficult (and far easier now than when I was first diagnosed), and the reward – being able to live a useful life for a normal span – is beyond price.

I don't want to give the impression that diabetes has dominated my life. Modern philosophers insist on the fluidity and multiplicity of identity, and 'diabetic' is only one strand in the skein that has been my experience. I have had three professions — academic, journalist and writer; I have travelled to many countries and lived in all three of the eastern Australian states; I have been twice married and a parent to three children.

So this is a very selective version that focuses on the diabetic strand rather than the others. I hope that this account of what I might call my diabetic life may help some people avoid the mistakes I made and tread a more intelligent and responsible path.

Peter Corris

Prologue

'WHAT THE BELL IS WRONG WITH ME?'

I rush down the corridor and take the steps four at a time, risking a broken leg, to get out of the school building and into the grounds. I spring for a tap, but not just any tap. This has to be the tap hidden around the corner from the quadrangle where everyone will be milling about in the midmorning break.

I reach the tap, turn it on hard and put my head under it. I swallow as fast as I can, gulping in the water, gasping for breath. It seems to take minutes before I can get enough water down to satisfy me. Then it's a dash for the toilet so that I can make it through the next two classes before my bladder bursts.

I hate myself. Why am I doing this? What the hell is wrong with me? *This is the third day. I think it* is some kind of moral weakness, like excessive masturbation. I know all about that. My mouth is dry within minutes of sitting down and thirst begins to torture me, although I must have drunk a gallon of water. I can't concentrate on the lesson. All I can think about is a running tap and how wonderful it would be to have my head under it with my mouth wide open. Now both weaknesses are clobbering me – the thirst *and* the bursting bladder. My skin is dry; I feel as if I am burning up but I am not sweating; I feel cold if anything, and weak and shaky. *Perhaps I am sick?* But I am rarely sick – the occasional cold or bout of flu – and I've never heard of a sickness that makes you drink like a fish and piss like a fountain.

Somehow, I get through to lunchtime. Another rush to the tap, then several long, gushing pisses during the 40-minute break. I wolf down my lunch of sandwiches and fruit and buy a pie and a drink at the tuckshop. I did this yesterday, too, and it is unusual because my pocket money is minimal and has to be made to last. I don't even like pies much but I want the bulk. The sweet drink doesn't do the job. Off to the tap again, and to the toilet. The afternoon session is a misery, but I manage to achieve the most important thing – concealing from my mates that anything is wrong.

The train ride from South Yarra – the station nearest Melbourne Boys High School – to my home station, takes about 40 minutes. Robert, one of my friends, is on the train with me. He gets off at Caulfield, four stations before mine, and I can hardly wait to see him go. I jump off the train at the next stop so I can piss and drink water, then I have to wait 20 minutes for another train. A leak at the station and a long, long drink and then the 10-minute walk home.

As I make the walk on a mild September afternoon, my schoolbag feels heavy, although there's nothing unusual in it, just the normal stuff for a night's homework and the novel I'm reading. I am an addicted novel reader, snatching pages whenever the opportunity presents, but I haven't opened the book for two days. Thirst and shame have been my companions. The bag is a dead weight and my limbs feel weak.

The dryness is on me again and I steel myself to act normally in front of my mother before I can get my mouth around a tap. Not for the first time, I notice how thin I am. I am ashamed of this, too. Ashamed of my chick-wing shoulder blades and scrawny chest. 'You're only sixteen. You'll fill out,' people have told me but it doesn't seem to be happening. Instead, I seem to be getting thinner.

As I open the gate, I think of the last two nights. They were terrible. In the small room I share with my younger brother, I had lain awake feeling my throat get drier by the second. I drank the glass of water I'd taken to bed but it didn't touch the sides. I was up and down, processing water, half a dozen times, with the house all quiet and my brother sleeping soundly. I envied him. It seemed that no sooner had I got to sleep than the pressure in my bladder would build and I'd be up again. It is a small house with only two bedrooms. My sister occupies a sleep-out in the yard, but the toilet is on the back porch and I can flush it without waking anybody, or so I think.

I am almost in tears as I have to summon strength to push open the light gate. My throat is on fire. It's no use. I'll have to tell them something's wrong with me.

CHAPTER ONE
'DOES THIS MEAN I CAN'T GET MARRIED?'

diabetes mellitus: a disorder of carbohydrate metabolism in which sugars in the body are not oxidized to produce energy due to lack of the pancreatic hormone insulin

Concise Oxford Medical Dictionary

When I got home from school that afternoon my mother was probably in the garden. We had a standard quarter-acre block and my parents were very proud of their garden. It had cement paths and borders to all the flower beds, a few shrubs and several fruit trees in the back. There was a lot of grass, front and back, and it was my job to keep it cut close with a hand mower. My mother seemed to find plenty to do in the garden, as she did in the house. She weeded, pruned, replanted and sprayed, none of which held any interest for me.

We had moved from Yarraville, a working class, western suburb of Melbourne, to Bentleigh in the south-east. Bentleigh was comparatively new. The area had formerly been known for its market gardens but the post-war suburban sprawl had engulfed it. Brick veneer was the dominant building style, and most of the residents, like my parents, were trying to better themselves.

I used the toilet when I got to the back porch, stumbled into the kitchen, drank glass after glass of water and dragged myself into my bedroom; no high-jumping or weight-lifting or tennis-ball-hitting this afternoon. No homework, either. I pulled off the hated grey suit jacket and tie, collapsed onto my bed and fell asleep.

My father was in the bedroom, looking concerned, when I woke up. It was rare for him to come into the room. Working and lower-middle-class

1

families in those days were extraordinarily prudish – I never saw my parents naked – and bedrooms were off-limits.

But here he was, sitting on my brother's bed looking worried. He told me that they had seen what was happening to me and they'd made an appointment for me to see the family doctor that evening.

'I can't stop drinking and going to the toilet,' I said.

He told me that when he was young and working some distance from home in a factory, he'd had a similar difficulty and had to wear a truss for a time to relieve the problem. He was no doubt trying to comfort me, but I couldn't see much connection between my plight and his.

After dinner my father drove me to the doctor in his old Vauxhall soft-top. I doubted I could have walked the mile to the surgery.

Dr John Storey was a typical family physician of the period – affable, over-weight and overworked. He chain-smoked Craven A cork-tips and nobody thought anything about it. His bulging waistcoat was always ash-streaked. Exercise would have been unknown to him, and his diet would have been like my father's – bacon and eggs for breakfast and red meat for the evening meal, seven nights a week. Both he and my father died in their fifties from heart disease.

We sat in the surgery, waiting our turn. My father's dry sense of humour often amused me, but there was always a distance between us. This must've been partly my fault; I was introspective and withdrawn, not a sunny youth. But I suspect that he was disappointed in me. He was a skilled carpenter, plumber and mechanic and I had none of these abilities and no interest in them. We had little in common and I didn't find conversation with him easy. That night, he probably looked at the magazines.

Appointment times with Dr Storey didn't mean much. If he felt like a chat with a congenial patient – about books, politics, religion – he'd have it, and the other patients could wait. I had seen the doctor off and on for minor things over the years – a bit of asthma when very young, a touch of bronchi-tis, eczema, a boil. Normally, I'd have taken a library book with me to read while waiting, but things weren't normal.

In what I later saw as a remarkable piece of serendipity, I picked up a copy of *Reader's Digest* and flicked through it, looking for sporting articles and checking to see if the condensed book was of interest. My favourite sections were 'Humour in Uniform' (a Cold War exercise, although I didn't know it then), and 'My Most Unforgettable Character'. I read those and then my eye fell on another article with a title something like 'Do You Have Diabetes?' I have often thought of searching the *Reader's Digest* index for the exact title of the article, but given the random and ratty state of Dr Storey's magazines, the issue could have dated from the '40s or even earlier.

I looked at the article probably because I had heard of diabetes as something suffered by the American tennis players Bill Talbert and Ham Richardson, but I knew nothing about the causes, symptoms and consequences. A few paragraphs were enough to convince me that I was a diabetic. The symptoms for juvenile onset *diabetes mellitus* were raging thirst, hunger, excessive urination, loss of weight – spot on. The disease had been fatal until the mid-1920s when control, but not cure, was achieved through the injection of insulin, combined with a diet that measured carbohydrate intake.

The article stressed that diabetics could lead normal lives, although the talk of injections and weighing food for every meal didn't sound so normal. I was not alone – as much as one per cent of the American population was diagnosed as being diabetic and the true figure was probably higher. Apparently, the disease did not hit everybody like a thunderbolt the way it had me. Some people displayed the symptoms in less drastic form over time and went into a slow decline. The *Reader's Digest* was not a publication that shirked the issue – the downside of diabetes was an increased risk of heart disease, a high incidence of blindness and in males (the word struck a fear into my heart that remained with me for almost 40 years): *impotence*!

I knew what impotence was. Henry VIII suffered it through disease and self-indulgence, Jake Barnes (*The Sun Also Rises*) through injury, and sundry other characters in fiction through illness, weakness of character and sexual ambivalence. It was a scary word, suggestive of doubtful territory; I remember reading it and closing the magazine. It meant you couldn't, didn't it? But my masturbatory excesses suggested that I could. It was a very confusing and frightening moment and, through no fault of his, being a man of his time, my father was the very last person in the world to talk to about it.

We went into the surgery, sat down and my father elaborated on what he'd already told Dr Storey on the phone. I confirmed a detail or two and was given a plastic beaker to piss into.

'Just a sample,' Dr Storey said.

He knew, as I knew, that I could have filled the bloody thing 10 times over. In those days urine was tested for sugar by means of an eye-dropper, a test tube and a reagent tablet. The result was never in doubt – the sample must have turned a bright red.

I can't remember the conversation that followed. My mother has told me that my father wept after he brought me home, but no man in those days would display that sort of emotion to his son. My recollection is that it was all business – another medical appointment first thing in the morning, nothing more to eat that night, and assurances all round.

Quite how the early appointment with the endocrinologist, Dr H Pincus Taft, was organised for early the following morning, I don't know. Perhaps Dr Taft had an answering service that would respond to urgent cases referred by a GP. However it was contrived, I was in Dr Taft's rooms in Collins Street with my father at 8am and a bag had been packed for me. I was going to miss some school in the important fifth year because I was going to hospital.

Dr Taft was a stocky, olive-skinned man with a shiny bald head and Semitic features. He was possibly the most urbane and sophisticated man I had met up to that time. He radiated intelligence and charm and I felt immense confidence in him. Like many, perhaps most, doctors of the time, he smoked. He offered his silver cigarette case to my father, who refused.

'I gave it up 10 years ago.'

'I wish I could.' Dr Taft tapped his cigarette on the case before lighting it. 'How did you do it?'

'Stubbornness,' my father said, an answer that accurately summed up a key element of his personality.

Dr Taft explained that I would have to have insulin injections and follow a strict diet and that this had to begin at once. I was not told why, but I later realised that the high sugar and ketone levels in my system, the result of my pancreas having completely failed to produce insulin, constituted a real danger of coma and serious damage to my health. Remarkably, after the time that has passed, some of the details of this meeting – like Dr Taft's immaculate white shirt and dove-grey suit – are clear. There was talk of health insurance and there the Corris family was well-covered. My father was a lapsed Mason but still subscribed to the health insurance scheme of the Manchester Unity Independent Order of Oddfellows.

Dr Taft favoured the Bethesda Private Hospital in Richmond as a stabilisation base for his patients. How I got there I don't remember... possibly in the Vauxhall. It's likely that my father took a day off from his job in the furniture department of Myer's store in the city.

I was given a bed in a ward shared with three other patients. I hadn't been in hospital for over 10 years (a brief admittance as a scarlet fever patient was my only other experience), but I was not particularly alarmed by it. There was a locker for my clothes and a bedside cabinet for books and other items. I still had the raging thirst and the weakness. I don't remember, but I imagine that I drank, pissed and slept.

Early in the afternoon, the girl in the bed next to me was visited by her doctor. This is a puzzling memory... it seems unlikely that they would put males and females together in a ward, but as I have a distinct recollection of a girl a few years younger than myself injecting her doctor in the leg with water (as a training procedure directed at teaching her to inject herself), I assume boys and girls must have been lumped in together. I remember seeing the doctor's white hairless thigh – he must have worn very wide trousers, but then they did in those days.

Dr Taft arrived and introduced me to the bottles of insulin with the rubber membrane over the top and the glass and metal syringe with its two needles – one for drawing up the insulin and a shorter one for the injection. He showed me how to purse up the flesh of my inner thigh, slide the needle in and press the plunger home. I did it the first time without a hitch. I was not then, and never have been, physically courageous, but injecting myself has never troubled me. I have now done it perhaps 30,000 times and, as Ned Kelly said: 'I think no more of it than to drink a cup of tea.' This was lucky; in those days, before the less formidable-looking disposable syringes and injection pens became available, some diabetics found the act impossible and needed a visit from a district nurse every day.

I was shown a roneoed list of forbidden foods and those that could be eaten, with careful measurement of their sugar content. All cakes, sweets, ice cream etc were out. I was taught to think of food in terms of 'portions' of 10 grams of carbohydrate. Mercifully, it did not have to be weighed, but the measurement had to be precise – a slice of bread was two portions, a serving of potato was so much, carrot was so much and the same with peas. Beans, lettuce, tomato, cabbage and other such watery and uninteresting foods were 'free' – diabetics could eat as much of them as they pleased. My daily allowance was 22 portions – six for each meal, one in between and two at bedtime. The theory was that the constant amount of insulin being injected should balance against the carbohydrate consumed, adjusted to the amount of exercise taken. This balance, where the blood sugar was supposed to remain as close as possible to that of non-diabetics, was called 'control'.

Within hours of the first injection, the thirst and hunger and the constant need to urinate left me. By evening I began to feel a renewal of energy and the meal wasn't too bad. I was so relieved to be rid of the debilitating and humiliating symptoms that the prospect of having to inject myself every day for the rest of my life and never again being able to eat chocolate cake or drink Coca-Cola did not bother me.

Like all Australian children of that time, I had been brought up on a high-fat, high-sugar diet. Sweet things – lollies, biscuits, cakes – were considered treats: rewards for good behaviour or celebratory indulgences. I had never had a particularly sweet tooth, although I ate icing sugar from the packet with a spoon on a couple of occasions and had Xmas and Easter binges. Excessive sugar had begun to take a toll on my teeth, which contained many fillings, but I was not obsessed with sweetness. I felt I would get by.

The dietitian explained certain things and several of the nurses talked to me as they went about their business. Only one thing about the whole bloody business of diabetes really worried me, and the presence of a couple of young, good-looking nurses intensified my concern.

I had never discussed sex with my parents. I had attended a 'Father and Son' night with my father at school but the sanitised biological style of the slide show was ludicrous. The only nitty-gritty reference to the subject in my youth was my father once saying to me: 'Your mother says you're not as

clean in your habits as you might be.' (She, of course, washed my pyjamas.)
So there was no way to come at the subject that terrified me directly.

They came to visit me in the evening and, very manly and brave, I
showed them the syringe and needles and told them about the diet.

'Does this mean,' I said to them finally, 'that I can't get married?'

Chapter Two

HE WAS ONLY SIXTEEN...

Honour the work, let our motto remind us When courage weakens and stern grows the fight.

Melbourne Boys High School song

As a kid, fantasies of various kinds dominated my life. I was a swot who wanted to be a sportsman. In primary school I'd have gladly swapped my full marks for reading and writing for selection in the first 18 of the house football team. In my fantasies, I made that initial step, did well, and then was promoted to the school team.

It never happened; I languished in the thirds and fourths and scratch teams, well below the notice of those who selected the good players for higher things. Academic ability seemed to be doled out in inverse proportion to sporting talent; I never saw anyone, boy or man, deliver a stab pass better than Rusty Fenton, who couldn't pass a school test to save his life.

I was average, or thereabouts, at most sports and yearned to be better. I certainly put in the time and effort. In the football season, I played endlessly at kick-to-kick (Australian football, the only code of any significance in Melbourne at the time). We played in the schoolyard and in empty lots, paddocks that broke up the uniform rows of plain, working-class houses in the Yarraville street. Occasionally, I took a good mark and delivered an effective drop-kick, punt or stab-pass – the drop-punt unknown in those days – but not consistently. You had to be consistent to get a guernsey.

Given that, it is amazing that I once had fantasies of becoming World Welterweight Boxing Champion. I had a makeshift punching bag set up in my father's shed, and my uncle Phillip, who had been a preliminary fighter, took me to bouts at the old West Melbourne Stadium. I saw Dave Sands KO Al Bourke and cried a few weeks later when he died in a truck accident.

But a punching bag cannot hit back. A few bouts in the YMCA, culminating in one when I was struck on the nose and wept, put this fantasy to rest. However, I bet the kid who beat me hadn't *read* nearly as much about boxing as me. I bet he couldn't have named all the world heavyweight champions from John L Sullivan down to Rocky Marciano, the way I could.

So, pre-puberty, my fantasies were of sporting heroics. In books borrowed from municipal libraries, the YMCA library and the Athenaeum Library in Melbourne, I read about sports endlessly – boxing, cycling, cricket, football, tennis, athletics. And I 'tried out', as the Americans say, for all of them – with indifferent results. At sport, as a boy, I was a thinker who wanted to be a practitioner, a theorist who wanted actual success. I idolised John Coleman, Hec Hogan, Dave Sands and Russell Mockridge, and only much later came to consider the strange fact that all of them had died young.

Looking back, I can see the mechanics of it all. In the social group I belonged to, practical skills were rated above all others and intellectual talents (especially of boys) were not valued. I absorbed these values. A frustrated athlete, I compensated by learning everything possible about those who could 'do'.

I came closest to competence at tennis. The game suited my physique and my temperament: physically cautious. My father had played when young – how well I don't know – but he owned cream trousers and a racquet, so must have made some investment. My parents forked out from their limited resources for equipment and tennis lessons for my sister and me. From the age of eight or nine and for the next 10 years I spent Saturday and Sunday mornings on the red-brown *en-tout-cas* tennis courts of the Melbourne suburbs.

Thanks to Mr Strachan ('Mr' the only name I ever knew the teacher by), I had a strong flat serve and a convincing forehand. I was weak on the backhand side, good overhead, but shaky at the net. I played club tennis and house tennis at high school – still not making the school teams, where players like Colin Stubbs were on offer – and twice competed in the Victorian schoolboys' championships at Kooyong. I survived a round or two only at singles, but Tom Wild and I progressed a bit further in the doubles one year. Not to the finals, though.

Inspired by seeing John Landy and 'Chilla' Porter at the 1956 Olympics, I ran assiduously on the school grass tracks and jumped into the shallow sandpits. I set up a makeshift high-jump stand in the backyard and once cleared five feet with a scissors Jump. The height has to be regarded as suspect. I hit tennis balls against the back wall of the house until I was ordered to stop because of the wear and tear on the grass. Anxious about my lack of muscularity, I made weights by filling jam tins and oil cans with cement and joining them with a length of water pipe. I lifted and pumped until everything hurt, with no noticeable improvement in muscle tone.

The only things that came easily to me were reading and writing. I continued to be a good performer in the classroom and at examinations, especially after the Intermediate when I was able to drop Maths and Science and concentrate on the humanities subjects that suited me. Several of my high school contemporaries have achieved distinction in academia and the law and I was on a par with them, or very nearly. I also regularly scored in the nineties for History; life in Bentleigh was dull – the past was glamorous and exciting.

But Melbourne Boys High School, excellent place of learning and sporting arena that it was, had one great drawback – no girls. I had kissed a few girls in primary school but none since. I was strongly attracted to females of all colourings and contours but painfully shy. My sex life was in my head and my hand – since the age of 13 or 14 I'd masturbated to fantasies... Brigitte Bardot in *And God Created Woman*, photographs of naked native women in the *National Geographic,* steamy scenes from the historical novels of Jean Plaidy and others.

Social tennis should have smoothed my sexual path. After a growth spurt in 1958, my sixteenth year, I stood almost six feet tall. I was not much afflicted by acne; I had thick, blondish hair, straight teeth and I tanned readily in summer. All around me my contemporaries were getting sexual experience through tennis – at dances, parties, film nights (television was only two years old, video was 21 years away, and the only way to see Wimbledon and the French and US Opens was on film), and trips to the country. My shyness was less acute when on a court playing mixed doubles.

At 16, I felt I was on the brink. Then diabetes hit me.

CHAPTER THREE

HYPODERMICS AND 'HYPOS'

'I fought Sugar Ray Robinson so many times I shoulda got diabetes.'
— **middleweight boxing champion Jake La Motta**

Diabetics diagnosed within the last 20 years would find the technology we used in the 1950s and 1960s like something out of the Stone Age. Instead of light, disposable plastic syringes, sealed swabs and pen injectors, we stored our glass and metal syringes and three needles (one for drawing up the insulin, one for injecting and a spare) in screwtop plastic containers filled with surgical spirit. Swabbing was done with cotton wool and methylated spirits – a bottle to be kept filled, more accessories not to run out of – but the spirit became milky after a time and had to be changed. The needles and syringes had to be sterilised each week by boiling, a tiresome task for a teenager.

Even more cumbersome was the equipment for testing the sugar level. The most common method was the urine test already described. Another plastic container held the test tube, eye dropper and reagent tablets. The kit came with a chart for recording the results of each test. The chart was submitted to the endocrinologist periodically for review of one's 'control', a fiddly, boring procedure. I am sure I was not the only young diabetic to lie about it – to tell my parents I had tested when I had not, to neglect to enter the results or to falsify them. Still worse, urine testing did not really work.

The major breakthrough in the treatment of diabetes came in the mid-1970s with the availability of the glucometer – a computerised machine that enables diabetics to accurately test their blood glucose levels.

Endocrinologists now admit that before the introduction of the glucometer there was no such thing as good 'control'. Some fortunate individuals were able to maintain near-normal blood sugar and have this more or less confirmed by urine testing, but for most it was a hit-and-miss affair.[2]

I spent several days in the hospital getting used to the routines of injecting, testing, maintaining the equipment and assessing the carbohydrate content of my food. This was to continue for a while at home but, fortunately, the September holidays were close and I would not miss much school. I enjoyed one aspect of my condition – being made a fuss of – but there was still the shadow of sexual inadequacy hanging over me.

I later learned that vascular damage of all kinds was thought to be an inevitable consequence of diabetes, however supposedly good the 'control'. This seemed to be confirmed by the observation that diabetics with good control suffered such damage, as well as those who were listed as 'uncontrolled'. Again, this was because the control was an illusion.

Despite the much publicised athletic successes of Talbert and Richardson and the intellectual achievements of such diabetics as H G Wells, there was a public perception of the diabetic as a frail, flawed creature. This was brought home sharply to me early in the '60s in the film *Hud*. In one scene Paul Newman is trying to placate the husband he has just cuckolded: 'Now Joe, you know you've got sugar diabetes.'

No fun to be cast as the cuckold rather than the stud.

Like any other Australian pagan I enjoyed a lie-in on weekends, but since the age of 16 I have not once 'slept in' in the morning: my day has begun with an insulin injection at approximately 7am.

I have developed a pattern where I get my deep sleep in the first stages and can readily wake up and function in the morning – a useful attribute and one of several things for which I have to thank diabetes. At first my mother had to call me at weekends but it soon became an ingrained habit and as a writer who likes to work in the morning, I came to value early starts in a quiet house after a solitary breakfast.

It was during the holidays, and my adjustment to the diabetic routine, that I experienced my first 'hypo' – diabetic jargon for hypoglycaemia, a drastic fall in the blood sugar level causing heavy sweating, physical weakness and mental confusion. I don't remember being warned against these events but perhaps I was. The cause in my case was invariably over-exertion at some activity – lawn-mowing or sport – without taking some sugar to retain the balance.

I sat in a chair in the living room on a warm afternoon and felt very peculiar. I had never sweated like this before; it was soaking my clothes and dripping into my eyes. My vision was affected by that and something else... a kind of distancing tunnel vision that made close objects seem small and far away. My mother found me before the level dropped too low and mixed a sickly sugar and milk drink that brought me out of it. I have had many such episodes since, and my saviour has always been a woman.

The hypo alarmed my mother and increased her protectiveness (already pretty well-developed as a result of the asthma phase in my childhood). As always in my family, euphemism prevailed over directness, and hypos were called 'reactions', a milder word. My mother was meticulous about my diet, insisting I carry barley sugar and the 'Diabetic Card' with me at all times.

The card, complete with my name, address and telephone number, read: *I am a diabetic. If found behaving oddly please give me sugar. If I fail to respond call a doctor or an ambulance.* I carried it, wrapped in plastic (laminating had not been invented) for years until it fell apart. It was not for another 20 years that I 'behaved oddly' enough to cause a member of the public to deal with me as recommended, and by then I wasn't carrying the card.

Hypos did not trouble me, perhaps because the ones I experienced at this time were not severe. I can't remember the insulin dose I was on (a mixture of Regular and Isophane insulins), but the amount was not large and consequently the sugar-lowering effect was not cataclysmic. In fact, I rather enjoyed the shift and sharpening (as it seemed) in mental focus that occurred in the early stages of a hypo. Once I stared at an apricot tree in our back yard and felt amused that I could count the exact number of carbohydrate 'portions' represented by the fruit on the tree. Later I was to experience much more profound and even transcendental insights into the nature of things when my sugar dropped.

When I returned to school I was briefly the focus of some attention, chiefly to do with the injections. Ignorance about diabetes was then, and still is, common. Some of my schoolmates wrongly assumed the disease was caused by eating too much sugar. Others mistakenly thought it was a hereditary taint. Interest in me soon waned when I appeared unchanged apart from slowly gaining weight and 'filling out', as I had long wanted to do. No more impulse purchases at the tuck-shop, though: it was dry biscuits for snacks, healthy sandwiches, fruit juice and milk for drinks. I used to go on long bike rides, 10 miles or so, and it had been one of my great pleasures to have a milkshake at the halfway point. No more.

Although diabetes seemed not to change me outwardly, it was causing important changes psychologically and physiologically – in fact determining the shape and direction of my life.

The shyness and lack of self-confidence that had inhibited me sexually and socially, intensified. I had a feeling that my life was artificially maintained, that it might well be shortened by vascular disease, and the shadow of impotence hung over me as it was to do for much of my adult life.

Poorly controlled diabetes causes changes in eyesight and these began in my case almost at once. Within two years I would be wearing glasses to correct deficiencies in my long sight, and over that period I lost the acuity that is essential to good tennis. 'Watch the ball onto the racquet,' Mr Strachan had instructed us and, although it is all but impossible to do when playing at a high level, it is still good advice. When I couldn't see the ball clearly and anticipate its flight correctly (although I wasn't aware of the fact), my weak backhand became even weaker and I had less confidence at the net. My previously reliable serve went off because I could no longer judge the distance between net and service line. I could still hit a strong forehand, almost by instinct, but it wasn't enough.

Playing bad tennis is no fun and is certainly no way to attract girls. I found excuses not to play at the club and any hope I might have had of making some social and sexual strides through tennis fell away.

The tennis club had provided my only contact with females, apart from my mother and sister, since the age of 12. The southern suburbs of Melbourne were islands of alienation; we 'lived next door' to people but had no neighbours in the full sense of the word. School friends were males.

I passed through a post-pubescent phase when homosexual experimentation might have been likely, but the rigid macho code of the time, and my class and circumstances (it must have been different at boarding school), made such activity literally impossible. I do not imagine that I was alone in this dilemma; shy boys like me were locked *into* heterosexuality and locked *out* of it at the same time. It was not a comfortable place to be and I cowered in it.

Always bookish, I retreated more and more into the world of fiction, where everything was so much more exciting and vibrant than in the world around me. I discovered the crime novels of Dashiell Hammett and Raymond Chandler and learned to admire their laconic, tough heroes. I greatly appreciated Chandler's wit and found his books amusing as well as gripping. 'It was a blonde,' he wrote, 'a blonde to make a bishop kick a hole in a stained glass window.' I yearned after blondes and had no time for bishops or stained glass windows. Everything about Chandler's choice of words appealed to me and, much later, when I came to write detective novels myself, I at first imitated him slavishly.

Hemingway became a great favourite and I quickly acquired second-hand paperback copies of all his novels and story collections, which I still have. His heroes, I recognised, were troubled, but their troubles seemed much more interesting and exotic than mine. I read, and was disturbed by, F Scott Fitzgerald. His characters seemed too close in spirit to me. I preferred Hemingway, realists like Steinbeck and Sinclair Lewis, and romantics like Ion Idriess.

I improved as a scholar as I spent less time on sport. I got high marks across the board, especially in History and English, in the term exams, and easily passed all six subjects for the Leaving Certificate. At the beginning of the year I had applied for, and was awarded, a £50 bursary from the Victorian Education Department. My sister had left school at 15 and only the winning of the bursary enabled me to stay for the extra year.

There was no tradition of higher education in our family. There were no bookshelves in the house. Apart from my mother's library books, kept neatly on her bedside table, the only books were a set of encyclopaedias, the complete works of Henry Lawson and a picture book about the First World War, kept in a cupboard in the hall. Money was short. Children were expected to go out to work after obtaining respectable qualifications and to pay for their keep.

My parents' plan was for me to leave school without matriculating and attend a Primary Teacher's College. University was not even thought of and I would then have had only the vaguest idea of what a university was. I would have known more about Oxford, Cambridge and Yale from my reading than about the University of Melbourne – then the only university in the state. But the diabetes was a spanner in the works. At that time diabetics were not accepted into the State Public Service. The fear was probably of hypos in front of a class and the risk of burdening the pension scheme. So a teaching career was out.

An uncle suggested that advertising might be the direction for me to follow and during the last term I went to a couple of interviews at agencies seeking juniors. I mentioned this to some of my teachers, who expressed surprise that I was not going into the sixth form. My good performance in the final exams evidently attracted some attention. Melbourne High was proud of its academic record and was in an annual competition with the public schools (the word used in the English sense in Victoria) for results in the Matriculation examination. I was considered a candidate for First Class Honours in two History subjects, Geography and English, and efforts were made to keep me at school.

The headmaster was W M ('Bill') Woodfull, the former Australian test cricket captain, 'a preeminent leader of men', as cricket writer Ray Robinson said. He was an austere figure who drove an elegant grey MG saloon car and wore immaculate dark suits. The 'head' did no teaching and was only visible at assemblies or when punishment was being meted out. Two years before, when a prefect had reported me for some minor infringement, he had given me a dressing down and detention.

Shortly before the end of the school year, I was summoned into Mr Woodfull's presence.

He had been grey and stern the first time, every inch the Methodist minister's son. His thin lips and pale eyes behind the wire-rimmed spectacles rebuked me as I stood in front of his desk. This time I was invited to sit and his tone and manner were kindly. He said that my teachers thought I should be given the chance to matriculate and that there was an Old Boys' scholarship available, worth £60, which would also pay for books. He wrote a note to my parents. They were impressed, but my father was resistant to the idea that his six-foot son, who was going on for 17 years of age, should continue to be a schoolboy.

My parents were products of The Great Depression. Though neither had been out of work at the time, both had siblings who had been and both knew many people who had struggled and some who had gone under. Their fixation was security, which explains the preference for the teaching service for me and a large insurance office for my sister. To my father, the notion of education for its own sake had no meaning. I had already had three more years of schooling than him and had been offered jobs by advertising agencies; why look any further?

My mother, who had also left school after two years of secondary education and who had worked mainly in shops before marrying, was a reader. I suspect that she was impressed by the word 'matriculation' in the headmaster's note. She was somewhat socially ambitious, intensely protective of me, and had a broader vision of life's opportunities than my father. With some difficulty, she persuaded him to allow me to stay at school as a compensation for the misfortune that had befallen me. I was all for it. I wanted to put off entering the real world for as long as I possibly could.

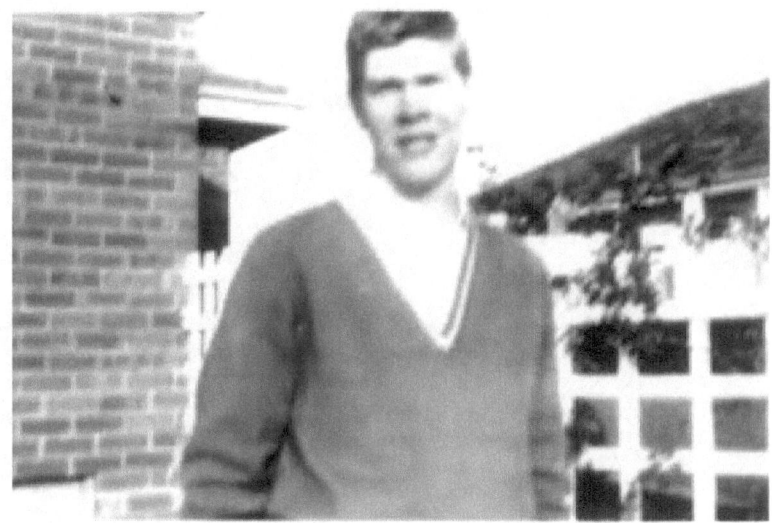

1.

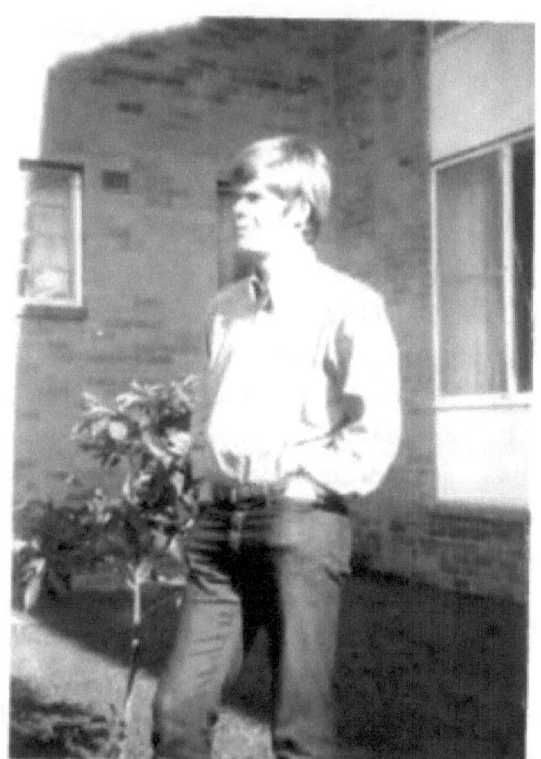

2.

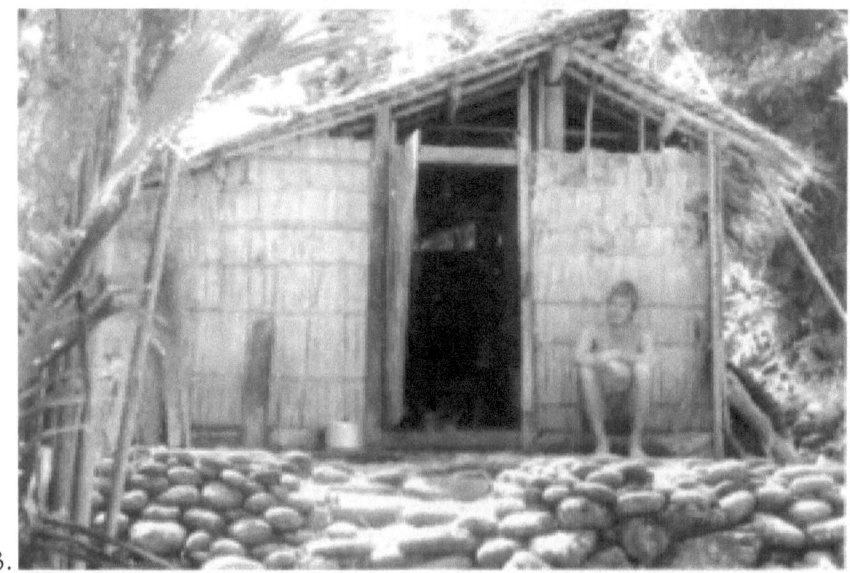

3.

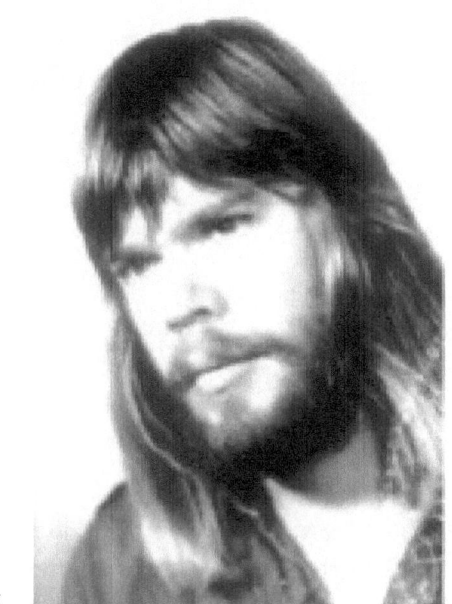

4.

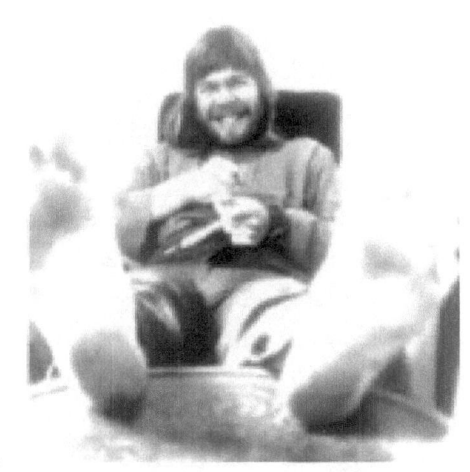

5.

Chapter Four
BAD HABITS

'Light up a Viscount, a Viscount, a Viscount Light up a Viscount, the best of them all...'

— **cigarette advertising jingle**

If I was to stay at school I was expected to work during the long vacation and contribute to the household expenses. At the end of my fifth year my father got me a job in the catering department of the Myer Emporium. The job involved unloading goods from trucks onto pallets and moving them up into the storeroom, squeezing oranges and taking the juice to the various bars around the store, taking chickens from the fifth-floor kitchen ovens to the rotisseries on the ground floor, and occasional stints cleaning up in the cafeteria and washing dishes.

I hated every minute of it and the pay was lousy – initially, from memory, £6.6 per week. I carried a paperback in my overalls and read during my breaks and illicitly snatched moments, trying to blot out the unpleasant reality.

There was a considerable amount of dishonesty all around – pilfering from the storeroom, watering-down of the coffee, adulteration of the 'fresh' orange juice with tinned extract. The rotisserie chicken counters were an outright scam. A few birds would turn on the spit inside a well-lit machine and finally be sold to lucky customers, but the great majority were cooked in fat up in the ovens, taken down and kept warm under the rotisserie and sold as the real thing. I knew, because I ladled the fat into the long trays, spiked the chickens to test whether they were cooked, prised them out of the grease if they had sat there too long and transported them on a trolley. People must have seen me unloading the chickens and taking away dirty trays but no customer ever protested.

In some ways the job was well suited to a diabetic. There was never any shortage of sugar around in case of a hypo. I had several as a result of working hard in a thick overall in the hot conditions but, of course, told no-one. We catering workers could eat very cheaply in the staff cafeteria, so there was abundant temptation. But I resisted – at that time I was a 'good' diabetic.

The only interesting thing about the job was the people I worked with. The store manager was Fred Taylor, obese and good-hearted, who treated his underlings well and was tolerant of my occasional need to take barley sugar and sit down for a rest. We talked football and cricket and films. He went to see the movie epic *Ben-Hur* soon after I had seen it.

'What did you think of it, Mr Taylor?'

He shook his head. 'Them Romans was a cruel mob.'

His 2-I-C was a Mrs Moir, a handsome middle-aged woman who wore her greying hair in a bun. Her manner was kindly, her smock was pink, her figure was good and I had fantasies about kissing her behind the shelves in the storeroom. I never did.

The catering staff were a mixed bunch. There were several trolley-pushers who were distinctly intellectually handicapped and some who were expert shop-lifters and passers of goods – hams, tinned food, sweets and biscuits in bulk – to accomplices who took them out of the store. I turned a blind eye to the lurks but was too cowardly to participate in them.

Myers employed many migrants (or 'New Australians') who worked hard and were generally honest. A Lebanese kitchenhand tried to seduce me in the changing room, but I was shy and scarcely aware of what he meant.

From time to time I bought lottery tickets, hoping for a win that would release me from the boring job, but with no luck. I got up at seven, took my insulin, had breakfast, caught the train into the city with my father, worked from nine to 5.30 (nine to 12.00 on Saturdays) six days a week, and had a day and a half off before the dreary routine began again. I played a bit of tennis, read books, went to the beach and yearned to be back at school.

I sometimes travelled home with my father and saw how tired and stressed he was. The vacation job confirmed my belief that the real world was tedious and hateful.

With my scholarship money making a minor contribution, I went back to school and into the sixth form, studying English, British History, Modern History, Geography (which qualified for matriculating purposes as a science) and French. Only French gave me trouble; the others were a joy. In that year I discovered the real pleasures of the scholarly life. This was just as well because I had no life or pleasure of any other kind.

I worked hard and Mr Munday, the British History teacher, had high hopes for me. Ben (as we all called him, but never to his face) was a short, overweight round-faced man with a snarling voice and a crooked grin. Nothing about his appearance suggested his intellectual calibre; his was an aggressive, competitive nature and he saw the British History examination as a sort of boxing match to be won by one of his fighters. Mostly, he trained the Exhibition winner (the student who topped the state) and he did so in my year. He encouraged me to think of going to Melbourne University to become a secondary school teacher.

'The Education Department won't have me because I'm a diabetic,' I said.

'You could teach in the public schools.'

Now *that* was a thought, but one I kept to myself. I couldn't see my father agreeing to me being a student for another four years.

I played less sport than before because I was studying hard and because my tennis was now so bad. The only compensation from the diabetes was that I was excused from the cross-country run in 1959. This event, conducted towards the end of second term, involved a five-mile (eight kilometre) run along the banks of the Yarra. I was reasonably fast over distances up to 880 yards (a little over 800 metres) but hopeless after that. I hated the crosscountry and seized the opportunity to duck it. The sports master was obliging because a student had dropped dead from heart failure the year before and the school did not want a repetition. This was the first time I used my disease to my advantage – malingered, you might say.

I stopped being a model schoolboy in the sixth form; until then I had been a complete conformist. I had enjoyed and taken such comfort in school that it had not occurred to me to question the rules. Now I did.

Then, as now, I hated choral singing. I absented myself from the compulsory practice sessions and nicked off from the house choral contest, held in the Melbourne Town Hall, by ducking into an arcade as we trooped up from Flinders Street station. I also used to wag it from Wednesday afternoon sport. Never good at or interested in swimming, I shot through from the house and inter-school contests.

On one of these escapades I was discovered, along with a couple of other delinquents, in the smoking compartment of a train, not wearing my cap or tie – and smoking. Happily, the teacher, Graeme Worral (later a colleague at Monash University) was also nicking off and was himself a smoker, so he didn't report us.

That incident taught me that, given a little luck, rules could be disobeyed with impunity, and not all of those charged with enforcing them took them seriously. As I also felt myself to be 'different' – having to stick needles in my leg in order to live and not being allowed to eat cakes – in some sense I felt that not all rules applied to me.

I took up smoking in 1959 and smoked, off and on, for the next 17 years. It was an act of rebellion: my father, like many ex-smokers, was violently opposed to the habit and I took to it partly in defiance of him. While at school and on a meagre allowance, I could only afford the occasional packet of 10 Capstan cork tips, (the cheapest brand on the market) but to buy and smoke them was still an assertion of independence from the house rules. It's hard to visualise now, but in those days, anyone big enough to get his or her money on the counter and state the brand could buy cigarettes.

The only recognised risk of smoking then was 'it will stunt your growth'. Already close to six feet tall, I had no worries on that score. In contrast to today's sports stars doing sincere anti-smoking advertisements, in the '50s they endorsed tobacco products, happy for their pictures to be on cards enclosed in cigarette packets. Footballers and cricketers were photographed with cigarettes to their lips, and no young Melbourne VFL supporter had any doubts why star South Melbourne forward Ron 'Smokey' Clegg was so nicknamed.

In any case, my fantasies of fighting for the World Welterweight Championship, of clearing seven feet in the high jump or playing Davis Cup for Australia were long, long behind me. I would be a physically flawed sophisticate, a cigarette smoker, a wearer of single-breasted suits, a schoolteacher.

CHAPTER FIVE

SIX QUID A WEEK

For Value & Friendly Service

— motto of the Myer Emporium

Haemophiliacs and epileptics, I assume, can forget about their illnesses for decent stretches of time. Not so the diabetic. Although the disease is less troublesome than epilepsy and less life-threatening than haemophilia, it is *there* all the time.

The day begins with insulin and thereafter every mouthful of food and drink is a reminder of the condition. And, since diabetics must eat something at about three-hour intervals through the waking day, and most take two or more daily injections, the reminders are constant. I am told by Dr Gordon Ennis, a former partner of Dr Taft's, that in Finland, where the incidence of *diabetes mellitis* is high, some diabetics take six injections a day in an effort to get closer to the natural process of secretion from the pancreas. I now take three injections and it wouldn't trouble me greatly to take six if better control resulted.

In the 1950s, however, one injection was the rule; the aim was to make managing the disease as comfortable as possible, and this was assumed to mean a minimum of injections. It was a serious misjudgment and many diabetics who went blind and died young could have been saved by a different injection regimen. I have to think that they would gladly have pricked themselves more often to save their sight and lives.

Ideas about diet, too, were unsound. While it was beneficial to avoid sweets, cakes, puddings and the like, there was too much emphasis on 'free' food – being able to eat as much meat, cheese, butter and eggs as you liked.

Many diabetic arteries, already adversely affected by the condition, must have been blocked solid by ingested fats.

From the age of 16 I ate no sugar and (in that pre-fluoride era) my teeth were relatively well-preserved as a result. I ate more fruit and vegetables than the average Australian, which was good, but too much animal fat – it was only by a lucky chance of genetic inheritance that I retained low cholesterol levels until the 1980s, when some real understanding of good diet came to the fore.

From the start, the dietary restrictions did not bother me much although I always felt free to interpret them in my own fashion. After the period in hospital and the spell at home getting used to things, my first venture out into the 'dangerous' world (my mother was nervous that I might 'hypo' getting off a train, crossing a road etc) was with my sister to see a film at a matinee session. I remember thinking *High School Confidential*, with Russ Tamblyn, John Drew Barrymore and the unforgettable Mamie Van Doren, was a pretty dopey picture, but I liked the Jerry Lee Lewis title song. At interval – my 'afternoon portion' time – I had a single scoop of vanilla ice cream, as was permitted. I also ate the cone, which wasn't.

My mother invested a lot of effort and expense to make my food as palatable as possible. At that time, a meal consisted of a main course and a dessert. Consequently, my mother bought 'diabetic jellies', 'diabetic puddings', 'diabetic jams' and the like, all sweetened with saccharine and generally nasty.

Saccharine tablets were used to sweeten tea and coffee but I disliked the after-taste. Later, artificial sweeteners improved but I soon acquired the taste for unsweetened hot drinks.

The worst of all these products were the diabetic soft drinks manufactured solely by the Boon Spa Company. My uncle, Neil Barton, a returned soldier whom I greatly admired for his good humour, sporting ability and confidence, arrived one day with a crate of these artificially sweetened 'aerated waters'. (There were diabetics in his family so he knew a thing or two about the disease.) It was kind of him, but the cola and lime and lemonade were horrible, and I never took to them.

Uncle Neil was fond of a drink and I heard that he said of me at the time: 'Poor little bugger won't ever be able to go into a pub and have a beer.' Little did he know.

In social terms, if not in technological ones, it was easier to be a teenage diabetic in the '50s than in the '90s. I knew no-one who drove a car and we gangly youths still rode bicycles everywhere, so I got the exercise necessary for diabetic control.

Diet-wise, there were fewer temptations then than now. The fast-food 'outfalls' (as Andrew Denton calls them), were in the future and the range of ethnic restaurants on display today would have seemed like a fantasy. The only non-Anglo-Celtic eating for the working class was done in Chinese restaurants, and I was instructed to steer clear of these because the cooks used sugar and honey in the sauces and dishes. When I did finally venture boldly and defiantly into a suburban Chinese restaurant in the early '60s I found the food disgusting and was not encouraged to try again for some time. I knew nothing about the fine eating houses in Melbourne's Chinatown.

In September 1959, aged almost 17-and-a-half, I had my first anniversary as a diabetic. I would have seen Dr Taft perhaps four times in the year and my report was good. I was filling in my test sheets in a desultory (and somewhat fraudulent) fashion, breaking my diet in minor ways from time to time, but basically still being a good diabetic. I was uninterested when told that a young woman who had lived next door had become diabetic during pregnancy. I felt no solidarity with other diabetics apart from the tennis players Bill Talbert and Ham Richardson, and that association was fast fading.

The Matriculation examination was the crucial rite of passage for academically inclined kids. As it was conducted in the heat of November and December, in an unfamiliar place with tension running high, there was an increased risk of hypoglycaemia.

By this time I had worked out that my emotional state, whether elation or depression, had an effect on blood glucose – but there was no way to do anything about it. Normally, I enjoyed examinations (except for French and Maths) and felt a quiet confidence, neither elation nor distress. But these exams might be different. I didn't notify a 'bulldog' (an invigilator – teachers earning a few extra quid) about my diabetes because, in those days, medical conditions were not taken into consideration. You sat the exam on the appointed day – sick, well or having your period – and that was that.

I went off with my diabetic card and barley sugar in my pocket. At that time, public examinations still had a distinctly nineteenth-century feel. For the humanities subjects, nothing could be taken into the room except a pen. You sat in a huge hall with hundreds of other candidates and everything was designed to run like clockwork. The question papers were already on the desks, with the candidates' number, but they could not be turned over and read until the head 'bulldog' said so. Also provided were lined booklets, one side of the page only to be written on. Absolute silence was insisted upon and any attempt to communicate with another student brought instant disqualification.

The bulldogs were formidable figures. Wearing academic gowns and stern expressions, they paraded up and down between the desks, continually trying to spot smuggled notes or coded information written on palms. All movement was suspicious. If you dropped something, you had to signal your intention to pick it up and were watched closely. Anyone wishing to go to the toilet had to ask permission and be accompanied by an invigilator. A warning buzzer was sounded 10 minutes before the end of the exam and when the final buzzer sounded it was pens down instantly.

I had no trouble with hypos until the Geography paper. The day was very hot and I was late leaving home. I ran for my train, just made it, but it stopped for what seemed like an hour outside Richmond station and was late getting into Flinders Street. I ran for the tram and then ran from the stop through the gardens to the Exhibition Building, arriving puffed and distressed and just in time to be one of the last permitted to enter the hall.

I should have realised something was wrong when it felt like a quarter of a mile walk to get to my seat. A distortion of spatial sense is one of the symptoms of hypoglycaemia. I was sweating, but the day was hot and I'd been running. (For no reason that I know, some diabetics have an inbuilt resistance to accepting that their blood sugar is low. I am one of them.)

I turned the paper over and ran my eyes down it, looking for the topics I'd studied and the way the questions were posed. I was a dab hand at twisting questions my way and making use of every scrap of information I had. The paper looked easy. But I couldn't get started. I fiddled and fumbled, dropped my pen and was cautioned for picking it up unbidden. I made a start on the first question and then found myself thinking about tackling the second while leaving the first unfinished.

This was nothing like my usual well-honed exam technique. Usually I allotted the appropriate amount of time to each question, finished within that span and left myself time for revision and polishing. I was alarmed by this departure from my tried-and-true method, and realised that I was having a hypo.

Fortunately – and surprisingly, given the prevailing puritanism – chewing was permitted in the exams. I dug into my pocket and shovelled my mouth full of the barley sugar, paper wrappings and all. I chewed and sucked and swallowed and felt the sweat dry and some clarity return. I'm not sure how much time I lost but it could have been half-an-hour out of the three hours. I soldiered on, making the best of it and not finding any snags in the wording of the questions.

Geography, as taught then, was mainly a matter of learning by rote how many frost-free days were required to grow maize; what landforms were created by vulcanicity and glaciation; what climatic pattern you had with average temperatures of X and average annual rainfall of Y. I had all this stuff at my fingertips and was very big on the river systems of the world and the characteristics of inland seas – still retained and useful these days for playing Trivial Pursuit against one of my daughters. I came out feeling that I had done pretty well.

The next day I was back in the hated white overall wheeling cooked chooks around in the Myer Emporium for six quid a week.

Chapter Six

GOING OFF THE RAILS

Claret is the liquor for boys, port for men, but he who aspires to be a hero must drink brandy.

— Samuel Johnson (J Boswell, *Tour to the Hebrides*)

The summer of 1959-60 is vivid in my memory. I hated the work in Myers, was in constant dispute with my father over such momentous matters as the width of trouser legs and the abilities of Elvis Presley, and was irked by the diabetic regimen. All novelty had long worn off and it was now a boring routine of insulin, testing my urine, avoiding hypos and eating dull meals.

I began to go again to the tennis club on Sunday morning (the more interesting and competitive Saturday session was out because of my job) and worked at my game. Forbidden the back wall of the house, I practised against a wall of the spectator stand near to the tennis courts. I read books about tennis technique, experimented with grips and ball tosses, but it was no use. My timing was off. By the end of that summer I had virtually given the game away.

As expected, Myers was a madhouse before Christmas. All floors were crammed with shoppers and the food counters did a roaring trade. I can't imagine how many fat-roasted chooks were sold as rotisserie chickens on Christmas Eve but it must have been thousands.

I earned extra money by working late that night cleaning up in the kitchen and at the point of sale. It was hot, heavy work, there was no air-conditioning, and the kitchens and service lifts and working areas were like furnaces. I ate extra through the day but still had a severe hypo in the service lift. I was in a bad way for a while with the barley sugar not doing the job, so

I grabbed and downed a bottle of Coca-Cola in the kitchen. I was astonished at how quickly the sugar-laden drink brought me to my senses.

Denied the sweets, chocolates, cakes etc that went with the festivities, I was something of an object of pity over Christmas. We celebrated in the English (Scottish?) fashion with a roasted turkey and all the trimmings at lunch ('dinner'), but there was no gravy for me. Gravy had flour in it and could not be accurately measured. There were no second helpings of roast potatoes, either.

The roast was followed by Christmas pudding my mother cooked in a cloth in the approved fashion and served with thick custard. The insertion of threepences and sixpences was still a feature because my brother was only 11 years old. I was denied the custard but not the pudding: in *Conquest,* the Diabetic Association magazine to which we subscribed (although I seldom read it), my mother had found a recipe for Christmas pudding with grated carrot for sweetness and substance. It sounds revolting, but was delicious – for me, the only pleasurable diabetic food.

And I suppose I drank the lousy Boon Spa cordials.

I did well in the Matriculation and, strangely enough, had my best result in Geography. I got a Commonwealth Scholarship which paid a small living allowance, and began an Arts degree at the University of Melbourne in 1960. Living at home, my mother prepared my meals and to some extent supervised other aspects of the diabetic life – testing, sterilisation of the equipment and so on. Though bored with the routines, I stuck to them.

After a successful first year, I changed to Honours in History and English, which involved a heavy work load and more time spent in the university library. I was still paying fairly strict attention to my diet but it was difficult to get the right amounts and combinations of food when eating out. However, towards the end of the year I began to stay at the university a couple of nights a week and eat in the cafeteria. My standard meal was a bowl of plain rice with an ice cream mashed into it. It actually tasted good and was exactly six portions. It was also all I could afford.

I learned that if I lived away from home I could get the full living allowance – enough to pay the fees at a residential college. Cameron Hazlehurst, a fellow

Melbourne High student who had duly won the British Exhibition at the matriculation exams and was on his way to a brilliant first class Honours degree in History and Politics, told me I could get into Ormond College. How I wanted to, but I didn't see how I could manage the food angle. Bloody diabetes.

With my first girlfriend at university I went to the first sub-titled film I'd ever seen: Resnais' *Hiroshima, Mon Amour*. We sat near the back for the obvious reason and I discovered that I couldn't read the sub-titles: they were a blur. Three years of imperfectly controlled diabetes had taken a toll on my eyesight.

This had a positive result. I was prescribed glasses to correct the damage, and my tennis improved. For the next 10 years I was able to play a respectable social game.

This first serious relationship was threatened when my girlfriend's parents expressed hostility towards me on account of my diabetes. They entertained some false ideas about the disease, particularly that Type-1 diabetes is an inherited condition; not unnaturally, they didn't want their daughter saddled with an invalid.

I did well in my second and third years there and, like some of the other ambitious Honours students, began to think in terms of tutorships and post-graduate scholarships leading to higher degrees. Diabetes was no barrier here.

In my final year I began to play fast and loose with it. After a year of eating with friends, male and female, in the university colleges and occasionally in hangouts such as Gina's in Carlton, I was more relaxed about guessing the carbohydrate value of food set before me. I didn't actually break my diet, eat cakes etc – but if a Gina's crumbed *cotaletta* with dressed salad and chips, eaten with like-minded, ambitious History students, resulted in a high urine reading that night, what the hell? I had enjoyed the meal and the company and things could be set right the next day.

Late in first term, I went to a History Department sherry party held in the Jessie Webb Library, a sacrosanct area reserved for Honours students, post-graduates and staff. The purpose, I suspect, was to look the final year Honours batch over as prospects for tutorships and post-graduate awards. I knew from novels that dry sherry was the right choice and as 'dry' signified 'not sweet', it was therefore OK for diabetics.

I was surprised to find how much I liked it and how it relaxed me. I chatted with Professor RM 'Max' Crawford, the Chair of the department who exuded Oxbridge sophistication and charm. Professor John La Nauze – 'Jack the Knife' – was harder going, but the sherry helped. I had never had such a good time in a social setting or performed, I felt, so well.

This was the beginning of a dependency on alcohol which has ebbed and flowed and plays a part in my life even today. A few days after the sherry party I made my first venture into a pub in Grattan Street, opposite the university. I did not even know what to ask for and, pretending not to speak English well, I communicated by gesture that I wanted a beer.

'A glass, mate?'

'Yes, a glass.'

I remember the taste of that first seven-ounce glass of fresh beer to this day. Like all kids, I had sampled the dregs at adult gatherings and found the stale, flat taste unappealing. This was different – this was magic, and I quickly learned the language: a pony, a glass and a pot.

It was madness. The sugar content of full-strength beer was high and I drank it freely over the next 10 years. I must scarcely have had well-controlled diabetes for 24 hours during that time and I was to pay a high price for the indulgence. Meantime, however, there was the instant dividend of sociability and confidence – two things I had lacked all my life.

1 went to the pub with fellow students and the staff members who drank – that is, almost all of them. I continued to work hard and spent Saturdays in the university library or the Victorian State Library, but I always had a drink or two afterwards. I remember getting into a discussion after a tutorial with Evan Jones, a poet and lecturer in English, about boxing. It was a mutual interest rare among academics, but he told me that Yvor Winters, an American poet and critic whom I admired, was a boxing fan.

We went to the pub and talked over many beers. I had a high capacity for alcohol and got only mildly drunk, but I forgot to eat and had a severe hypo on the train on the way home. The barley sugar pulled me out of it, but only just. I rinsed my mouth at the front garden tap and crept into the house. My parents knew nothing of my new life.

I was playing tennis fairly regularly at the club and with university friends. The walk to the train station was almost a mile and I sometimes walked from Flinders Street station up to the university, another mile or more, to save on the tram fare. I suppose that all this activity compensated to some degree for the ill-judged meals and the beer, as I felt strong and well.

Chapter Seven

SEX IN THE SIXTIES

Sexual intercourse began
In nineteen sixty-three
(Which was rather late for me)
Between the end of the Chatterley ban
And the Beatles' first LP

— **Philip Larkin, *Annus Mirabilis***

Towards the end of second term in my final year I went to the annual history conference at a guest house in the Dandenongs, near Warburton. Conferences were opportunities for Honours students to strut their stuff by giving papers on various subjects – a bit earlier I had gone to a similar English department conference and given a paper on de Lampedusa's *The Leopard* – and an excuse to get away from home and to have sex. Established student couples used them as dirty weekends and others among staff and students hoped to do the same.

I've forgotten the subject of my paper at the history conference, but I remember being introduced then to claret and edam cheese. Claret was dry wine I was told, sugar free, and I drank as much of it as I could afford. The cheese on biscuits I didn't bother to take into account for my diet.

I was still living at home and my mother saw to it that I kept to my diet there, but outside the house it was a different matter altogether. My parents were teetotallers and non-smokers, but I was now earning a little extra money by tutoring high school students in the evening, and away from home I was drinking regularly and demonstrating my sophistication by smoking Senior Service cigarettes. Wine, bought in tall Wynvale flagons, was good and inexpensive; compared to the price they are today, cigarettes were also very cheap.

At the conference, I shared a room with another student. One evening, probably emboldened by red wine, I playfully put my arms around a girl and bundled her into the room. Margaret Brown, whom I'd known slightly for about a year, was one of the leading lights of the History Honours group. She was the girlfriend of another history student and my assault on her was purely in fun. She didn't resist and we halfembraced before I stepped away, embarrassed at having almost made a pass at a mate's girlfriend.

To my surprise, Margaret rang me up a few days later and suggested we go out together, inevitably to a foreign film. I forget the title – I saw little of it. Margaret was tall and extremely handsome with magnificent brown hair and a slender, athletic figure. She and I had a good deal in common (and many differences, as it turned out).

Her family was working class, living in Seddon, the suburb next to Yarraville, where I'd spent my early years. We were both products of the selective high system, Margaret having gone to University High School and done brilliantly in the Matriculation and in her early years at the university. Similarly, we were at odds with our families over education, lifestyle and our ambitions. My family knew nothing about my academic aspirations while Margaret's people, who knew she was attending the Secondary Teacher's College, were unaware that this meant she was enrolled for an Arts degree at the university.

I was 21 and still a virgin. My last girlfriend had been a devout Anglican and chaste, while I was a convinced atheist. Our relationship had foundered on that difference (in fact she left me for a priest whom she ultimately married.) Margaret was agnostic and sexually vibrant and I fell in love with her. The fear of impotence that had haunted me for years was set aside.

After the final Honours examination in Far Eastern History, the lecturer in the subject, Dr Jack Gregory, took the small class out to a meal in Chinatown. This was my first experience of good Chinese food and, while I've never become a devotee, I found the atmosphere exotic and interesting. Margaret and I often ate Chinese and I often had high urine sugar tests as a result. I was too happy and foolish to care.

I topped the course in Combined History and English Honours and was appointed to a Teaching Fellowship at Monash University. John Morgan, the lecturer in the subject I taught (British Constitutional History) and I got on extremely well. I admired him, copied his habit of rolling his own cigarettes, and enjoyed many a dry sherry with him in his room at the end of the day. Then, long before breathalysers, half the university staff would have taken to the roads 'over the limit'.

John's wife, Trish, was from the Catholic squattocracy. She was dark, exotic-looking, very good company and a fine cook. Margaret and I often went to the Morgan's house for dinner, and on these occasions, I paid only lip service to diabetes, eating and drinking far too much and ignoring the urine test results. Or neglecting to test at all.

Newly affluent, I frequently ate in Carlton's Italian and French restaurants with the same carelessness. It was traditional for the staff to drink at the Notting Hill Hotel with the older students and I was an enthusiastic participant. I had virtually given up sport, drove everywhere and got no regular exercise – I was embarking on a lifestyle totally inappropriate for a diabetic and one that would eventually cost me dearly.

Daunting though my first try at lecturing at Monash was, it was nothing compared to a two-week bout of impotence I suffered during the year Margaret and I were engaged. The relationship was never tranquil; we quarrelled over various things and she several times called off the engagement, only to relent when I pleaded with her. Our lovemaking took place in the car, parked in deserted spots in the bitter Melbourne winter, and was increasingly unsatisfactory. Eventually I was in despair at being unable to perform and all my old fears resurfaced. I now know that anxiety about sexual performance stimulates the production of adrenalin, which constricts blood vessels and intensifies the problem. I knew nothing about such things then and felt that the bottom had dropped out of my world.

Margaret was patient and sympathetic and we decided to book into a motel to see if more comfortable surroundings and the aid of a bottle of wine – and no time constraints – might help matters. In the early 1960s this was a fairly bold move and took some hide to pull off. The motel receptionist clearly did not believe that we were married, as I claimed, but didn't comment. The whole episode veered towards farce when the car wouldn't start and had to be pushed from the check-in area to the room. We laughed, I relaxed, and the experiment was successful.

But the whole experience had damaged my new-found sexual confidence and I began to use alcohol to bolster what remained of it. This potentially dangerous strategy worked for quite some time.

My sexual fragility was due mainly to overextended virginity as well as to inexperience and ignorance. Foreplay was inadequate and ineffective; I knew nothing about oral sex, lubricants, massage oil and all the other devices and techniques to stimulate and maintain arousal and sensitivity. It is possible that five years of poorly controlled diabetes had begun to damage my vascular system just as the *Reader's Digest* article had outlined, but I gave no thought to this, and did not seek medical advice. When I suffered impotence my reaction was to panic and doubt my masculinity.

I got on well with Margaret's father, who for some reason called me 'Rooster', and who always had a bottle of Dietale in the fridge for me. Dietale was low-carbohydrate (but alcoholically full-strength) beer. It might have been possible to drink it judiciously and not disturb the 'control', but I was not judicious. I drank to excess – wine, beer and spirits – because I enjoyed the taste and the effect: a feeling of relaxation, an infusion of confidence, an antidote to shyness.

Margaret and I were married early in 1965 and, after completing a Master's degree during my three years at Monash, I won a scholarship to study for a Doctorate at the Australian National University, in Canberra.

After a gap of a few years, I consulted Dr Taft before leaving Melbourne. I did not tell him the truth about my way of life, but admitted that I was having difficulty with control, testing high and experiencing some hypos. He recommended that I change to two injections daily, mixing Semi-lente, a slowish-release insulin and Actrapid, a quick-acting variety, for the pre-breakfast dose, and Monotard, a slow-acting insulin, before the evening meal. This, an improvement on the old regimen, became my routine for almost the next 20 years.

As far as my diabetes was concerned, the move to Canberra was a disaster. I lost contact with Dr Taft, who had exercised some restraint over me in Melbourne; there, I would 'clean up my act' at least for some time before my visits to him, and take care of myself for a while afterwards.

In Canberra, I did not see an endocrinologist and my neglect of the disease grew worse. I became a heavy, regular drinker. Whereas previously I had periods of light drinking and days when I didn't drink at all, I now drank every day and often at lunch as well as after the day's work and on into the evening. Research scholars were eligible to become members of University House, a kind of residential college, where there was an excellent bar. I drank there often, usually beer and in excessive amounts, with Jim Davidson, the Professor of my department, Deryck Scarr, my supervisor, and others. One signed chits for drinks and my monthly bill read 'Bevs, Bevs, Bevs', and nothing else.

I injected twice a day, followed the diet in a rough and ready fashion (making no allowance for the beer) and tested the urine irregularly. The distance to the university was short but I drove in my new Volkswagen. I smoked. My only exercise was an occasional game of tennis with Margaret and friends (invariably followed by drinking), and some swimming in summer: not nearly enough. At this time, when the blood sugar must have been far too high most of the time, serious damage was being done to blood vessels in various parts of my body. I should have known about this but didn't. I felt well and was capable of working long hours and playing for just as long.

Margaret and I became friendly with several other couples living in the apartment block allocated for married students without children. We ate frequently in each others' flats, held parties and conducted marathon card and darts games. At that time you could buy spirits cheaply in two-litre flagons and we sometimes laid in quantities of gin, Tarax tonic water and lemons. We drank and smoked and threw darts from the afternoon into the evening and through to the early hours. It was great fun and I gave no thought to what the sweetened tonic water and hastily snatched meals could be doing to me.

CHAPTER EIGHT
PUNISHMENT IN THE PACIFIC

My first impression was of a place so ramshackle, so poor, so unexpectedly filthy, that I began to understand the theory behind culture shock... The idea that this miserable-looking town could be regarded as a capital city seemed laughable... *Why would anyone come here?*

Paul Theroux, on his first impressions of Honiara, capital of the Solomon Islands. (*The Happy Isles of Oceania* p148.)

Looking back, I should have asked Dr Taft to refer me to an endocrinologist: with the John Curtin School of Medical Research one of the major units of the University, there must certainly have been endocrinologists about. I should have located and joined a diabetic support group and kept abreast of developments in the treatment of the disease. I should not have smoked. I should have exercised regularly and kept strictly to my diet. Above all, I should have kept my alcohol consumption to a safe level.

Now, when I do most of these things, it seems remarkable to me that I did none of them back then.

There are no excuses for my neglect, but there are reasons, and one lies in the nature of diabetes itself.

Unlike a physical disability, it is not apparent to others and it is possible to conceal it. Whereas the effects on schizophrenics and epileptics of not taking their medication are obvious, this is not the case with diabetes. Someone neglecting the disease as I did will not necessarily suffer hypoglycaemic attacks, which would cause comment and maybe intervention, but is more likely to have continual high blood sugar readings which have no behavioural consequences.

If I had been less healthy, subject to illnesses or consulting doctors, I might have been advised to pay more attention to my condition. But I was very 'healthy' and only remember seeing a doctor once in my student days in Canberra. Above all, I believe I was ashamed of being diabetic.

The neglect was a way of denying it to myself and others. I showed that I could behave normally – that is, indulge in all the bad habits that undermine the health of Australian men. In my case, however, that undermining was rapid and serious.

My ignorance of diabetes was inexcusable. In 1961, one of my lecturers, who was also a diabetic, gave me a copy of *The Diabetic Life*. If I had read it I would have learned enough to warn me of the dangers of my lifestyle.

The book travelled with me to Canberra, but remained unopened.

My subject of study was the Pacific islands labour trade, a mass movement of indentured labourers who came from the Melanesian islands to Queensland, Fiji, Samoa and other places, to work on plantations. I concentrated on the Solomon Islands and in 1968 spent three months in Queensland interviewing descendants of the labourers, popularly known as 'kanakas' and calling themselves South Sea Islanders.

This involved travelling by rail, car and bus from town to town, and inevitably, much of my work was done in the pubs. We drank five-ounce 'ponies' (the beer got warm in bigger glasses), ate in cafes, restaurants and people's houses, and I only approximated to my diet. The work went well – I collected the information I needed – but my diabetic control was steadily slipping.

The following year I spent six months in the Solomon Islands and Fiji interviewing survivors of the labour trade. Diabetes was a decided handicap as it was not always possible to eat meals at the regular times demanded by the insulin injections, and the physical effort involved in this work could vary from near exhaustion one day to total idleness the next. I suffered many hypos, quickly used up my barley sugar supply, and had to buy packets of CSR sugar from the village stores (little more than cupboards stocked with tobacco, sugar, rice and canned goods) to see me through.

I tried to explain the condition to John, my local helper. He was a mission-educated youth, but the sight of the hypodermic terrified him and I dropped the subject.

One of the best indications of the onset of a hypo was sweating. In the Solomons I sweated all the time and often failed to detect the early warning.I often woke on a hot, steamy morning in a stifling hut drenched in sweat. At other times, when staying in towns, government rest houses or on plantations, my sugar would have been high. Oscillation from low to high levels is a bad situation for diabetics, scarcely better than having no treatment at all.

Mostly, I lived on yams, tinned fish, rice and bananas. Luckily, I have always liked bananas. Several times I ran out of fish and dined on boiled rice and tomato sauce. This isn't too bad once or twice, but palls pretty quickly.

The most congenial missions were those of the Marist Catholics, where alcohol and tobacco were available. At one point, after a particularly arduous passage by land and canoe and with my supplies exhausted, I staggered into a mission only to find that it was a Seventh Day Adventist hospital. Admirable, of course, but there was no tobacco to be had, no alcohol, and the evening meal I was so generously invited to share was based upon the soybean nut cutlet. I left the following day.

Usually, I travelled by government launch but sometimes by copra boat as a deck passenger, as there were no cabins. I returned in this from Ysabel in the north to Guadalcanal, through a storm so severe that all the deck passengers had to lash themselves together and to stanchions mounted on the deck. In reasonable conditions I was a good sailor, but this time we spent 12 hours amid the copra sacks in wringing-wet misery. I vomited almost continually and could neither eat nor take my insulin. I lost 10 pounds on the passage and could scarcely walk. My biochemistry must have been in a mess at the end of it.

Towards the end of my time in the Solomons, I made a trip to Marau Sound, no great distance from Honiara, to collect stories about an attack on a labour ship. A local planter put me up. He was like a Somerset Maugham character – totally hospitable, and immensely overweight to the point of immobility. Each morning he sat on the verandah drinking beer – he worked his way through most of a case in the daylight hours – and gave orders on the day's operations to his 'boss-boy'. For the rest of the day he drank, read paperback thrillers and slept.

I always travelled with a selection of paperbacks, mostly mysteries bought in Honiara, and the planter and I had a lively exchange of views on the various writers and the books themselves. I did my interviews and then had a few days to wait for a boat back to the capital.

I walked around the plantation (which provided the model for any subsequent writing I did on life in the tropics) and swam off the shingly beach. One day I happened to be wearing thongs instead of the usual sandshoes, and cut my foot on a piece of coral. I thought nothing of it and the cut rapidly became infected. I was feverish within 24 hours and a red line ran up my leg towards my groin from the swollen foot. The planter had no antibiotics and a severe infection plays havoc with sugar levels, the liver secreting glucose to enable the body to cope with the assault. To make matters worse, a storm blew up and the boat I was expecting to catch was delayed.

In one of the most frightening episodes in my life, I lay in bed and heard the planter receive instructions over the radio about how to anaesthetise me and amputate my leg to prevent my dying from gangrene. I was feverish and weak and couldn't have prevented this happening. Fortunately, the boat arrived and took me immediately to the hospital in Honiara. I received a massive – and very painful – injection of penicillin and was out of danger within a day. I sent the planter, who had spent hours at the radio monitoring the boat's progress and offering me encouragement, a bottle of the best Scotch whisky in the Burns Philp store.

CHAPTER NINE
WARNING SIGNS

warn: to tell or signal to a person that something, usually bad, is going to or may happen...

The Pocket Macquarie Dictionary

I completed the fieldwork without further mishap and returned to Canberra to write the thesis. Margaret had gone with me to the Solomons but had found the climate and conditions too trying and hadn't stayed. Our relationship had always been fragile and, now, after being apart for six months, it collapsed. She returned to Melbourne and I coped with my distress by working feverishly.

In 1969-70 I probably did more damage to my health than at any time before or since. I completed a draft of the thesis in six weeks and had almost a whole year to polish it. I submitted it to my supervisor in sections, pretending that I was working steadily; in fact, I was playing. With time on my hands, no responsibilities and sufficient money, I enjoyed myself.

I had a series of relationships with women around the university, went to parties, drank with other students and staff and visited Sydney for more of the same.

A very distressing episode of impotence around the middle of the year should have rung alarm bells. I saw a doctor who prescribed a mild sedative, I slept deeply for 24 hours and had no further sexual problem. Surely it was the responsibility of this doctor, confronted with a diabetic experiencing impotence, to question him closely about his control and insist on blood tests? Why didn't this happen? I doubt that I can blame the doctor – I probably didn't tell him I *was* a diabetic.

I was awarded the PhD and won an Australian National University Travelling Postdoctoral Fellowship. This provided enough money to enable me to travel overseas and pursue further research. The only requirement was that I submit a short report upon my return regarding the work I'd done. I planned to continue studying Pacific History in British archives, visit friends and other academics in Europe and the United States and do more research in Fiji.

Before leaving I had a brief time in Sydney where I conducted two sexual relationships, not very successfully. I had inherited a couple of thousand dollars from my uncle Philip (the one who'd taken me to the boxing) and spent a good deal of it on Quelltaler hock and at places like the superb Spanish restaurant, Costa Brava, and at the Newport Hotel where I passed on Sundays as a *bona fide* traveller.

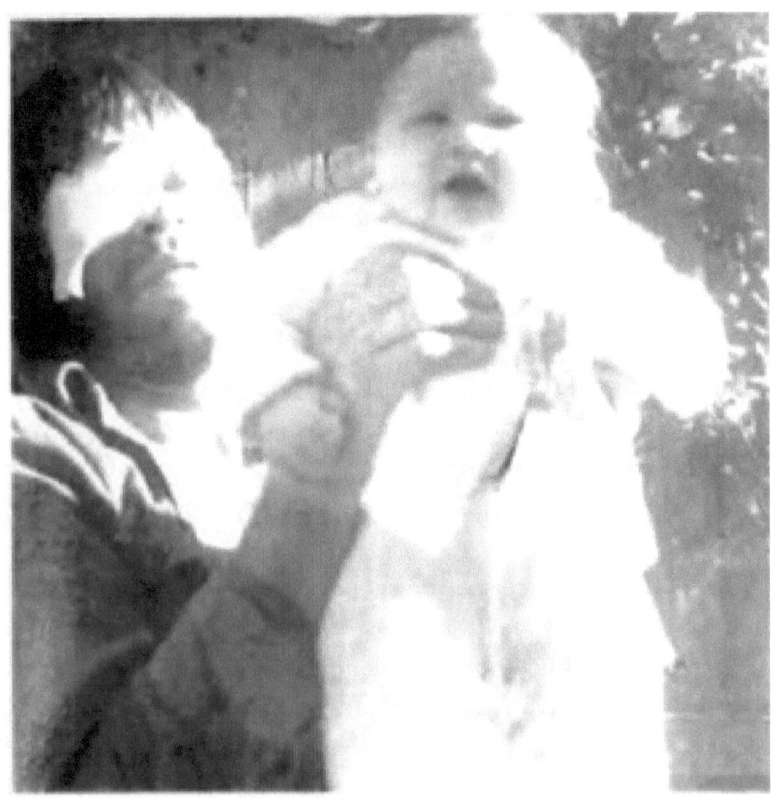

6.

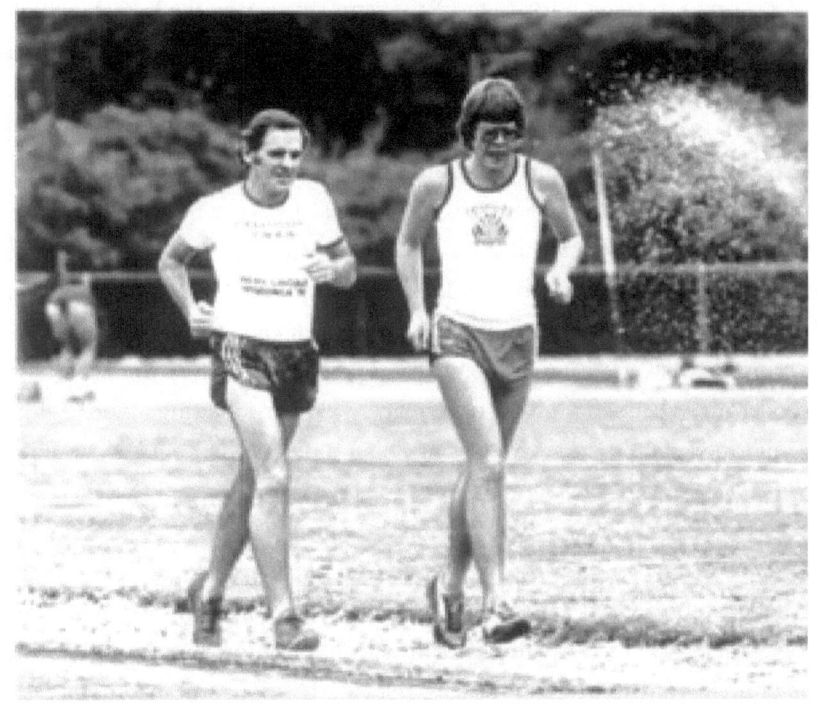

7.

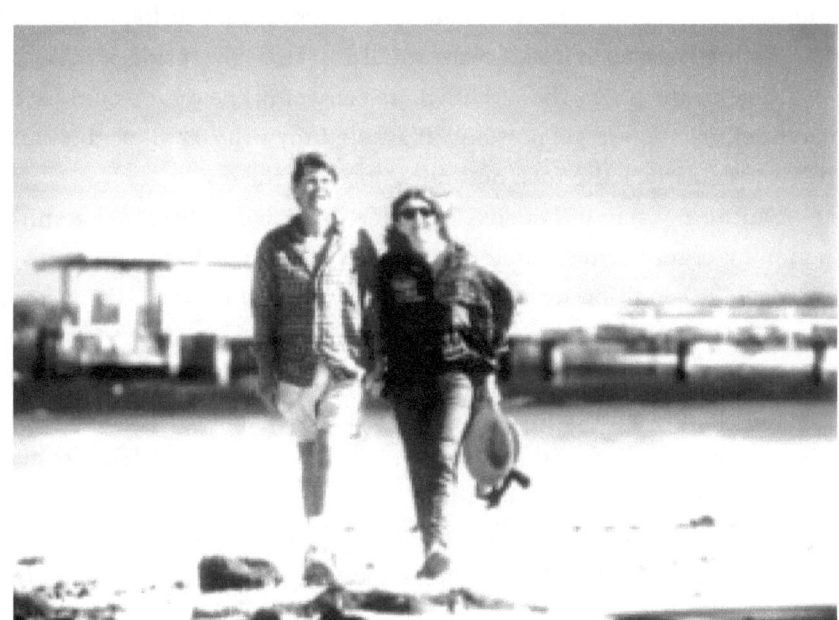

8.

I had short stopovers in India and Russia on the way to the UK. My passport photo from the time shows a typical hippie – shoulder length hair, beard, and an army disposal shirt.

After an interminable wait at the departure gate at Moscow airport, I presented my travel documents and duffel bag. The beard and the long hair were suspect and my bag was searched. The official found my syringe and needles and I was escorted to a small room, made to wait and was then questioned by someone who had virtually no English. The plane was due to take off soon and I dreaded missing it; I had already had more than enough of Russia. I regretted not carrying my diabetic card and found it impossible to convey the reason for the hypodermic. The bland, grey Russian faces were intimidating, and the number of uniformed pistol-packers wandering about didn't help. Eventually an English-speaker was located. I explained things to her and was allowed to leave.

While in England I began to keep a diary, but there is virtually no mention of diabetes in it. One entry recounts meeting up with John Morgan, then on sabbatical leave, and his family for lunch in a Guildford pub. I sat down to one of my favourite English meals – liver with onions, mashed potatoes, and Yorkshire pudding washed down with two pints of draught Guinness stout. The only reason I recorded what I ate was my amusement at John's comment.

'Eating that much iron, Corris, you'll rust from the inside out.'

More to the point, the carbohydrate content of the meal would have far exceeded my allowed six portions. If I tested my urine at all at this time, I did it irregularly. I also took not much notice of the results.

During my stay in London, I became ill with diarrhoea and vomiting: poisoning of some kind. Careless of my health as I was, I knew that this was a dangerous condition for a diabetic, and dragged myself to the doctor for treatment – under the National Health.

I recovered from the bout and when I returned for a checkup, the doctor suggested I could control my diabetes by oral medication rather than by injecting insulin. This was ignorant and irresponsible: Juvenile-onset diabetes cannot be controlled in this way.

But I was equally ignorant and tried the tablets for a week – a miserable failure, resulting in a return to thirst and slurping gallons of water. I had enough sense to revert quickly to insulin, but not enough sense to try to regain something approximating control.

As in my early student days, it's likely I kept the sugar levels under some rough restraint by walking great distances. London in 1970 was still swinging but I didn't have the confidence to swing. I spent a good deal of time on my own and killed much of it with the walking.

I covered a good deal of inner London, visiting the places I had read about – Bloomsbury, Hyde Park, Highgate Cemetery (to see the grave of Karl Marx), Hampstead Heath, Whitechapel (I was something of a Ripperologist), and went by train to Brighton and Hastings, where I also walked. I had occasional hypos, suggesting that the sugar level was not consistently high, but insidious damage was certainly being done. As always, I drank too much and smoked.

At that time smoking was permitted in cinemas. I went often to films in the city, Chelsea and Knightsbridge, smoking along with the rest.

Towards the end of my time in England, Jim Davidson, the professor in the department where I had done my doctorate, wrote and advised me to apply for the Research Fellowship in Pacific History currently advertised. I did so and received a telegram from him, telling me I had the job, subject to a medical examination.

I took steps to get my blood sugar down to acceptable levels. For a week before the medical I drank little, kept strictly to my diet, walked and tested regularly. The doctor who examined me was an extremely handsome woman, not much older than me. There was a minor glitch when an irregular heartbeat was detected, but I was able to convince her that this was a benign heart murmur, first diagnosed many years before. I characterised myself as an 'occasional social drinker' and a 'light smoker'. I passed the medical, although both my blood sugar level and blood pressure were higher than they should have been. The doctor also reported some deterioration of vision in my left eye.

Again, these would have been urgent warning signs to anyone with a knowledge of the downside of the disease. I should have investigated this further, questioned the young doctor closely and learned more. Should I have been issued warnings and advised to see an endocrinologist? Perhaps, but they were my eyes and I should have been seriously alarmed. In my ignorance I wasn't, and did nothing.

My companion at this time was a woman I'd met in Canberra. She came to England to stay and travel with me through the long Australian academic vacation. I had always minimised the importance of diabetes and she had no reason to think that our pub-going, exercise-free lifestyle was damaging. Her staples were Coca Cola, scotch whisky, cigarettes and potato chips – I can't recall her ever cooking a meal. While I ate more healthily than that, trying to include fruit and salad, if not fresh vegetables, my diet fell a long way short of what it should have been. We went to Ireland where, inevitably, I drank a lot of calorific, high carbohydrate draught Guinness.

When I look back on that time from 30 years later, I feel very little connection with the person I was then. Instead, I am inclined to analyse his actions and motives as I would those of a character in a novel. I am led to the conclusion that for that 28-year-old man, things were apparently going extremely well – far better than he could have expected. He had escaped the suburban dreariness, travelled, gained high qualifications, been appointed to a prestigious job, had a handsome and congenial companion and influential patrons, and a bright future.

Far from being a handicap, diabetes had been a springboard to a richer life. What reason was there to fear or pay much attention to it?

CHAPTER TEN
'BY THE WAY, HE'S A DIABETIC'

'A diabetic? Nothing but trouble. Don't have anything to do with him'.

Clare Golson to jean Bedford, 1972

After eight months in Britain and Europe, I travelled to the United States. It's clear from my diary that I was paying little attention to diabetes at this time; there is no mention of urine testing. The reagent tablets would have been very expensive in the United States without a prescription, so I have to conclude that I was not testing at all, just flying by the seat of my pants.

Likewise with diet. I recorded my experiments with American food: tacos, which I found uninteresting; grits (tasteless), and the palatable but high carbohydrate hash browns. I also ate in a McDonalds (then a fairly new phenomenon) but the hamburger was awful and the filling and bun insipid. I have never been inclined to repeat the experience.

On the credit side, while in New York and Boston, I was walking a good deal and eating plenty of delicious Californian fruit. Against that, I was drinking a lot of the very good and cheap Californian red wine (no-one drank white wine in those days).

I flew to the west coast to give a lecture at the University of California at Santa Cruz. I had shed the beard and looked much younger than my years. As the legal drinking age in California was 21, I was constantly being challenged as to my age when drinking in bars or buying wine and beer in supermarkets. I carried my passport with me at all times. Although I was frequently asked by teenagers to buy beer for them, the penalties for doing this were severe and I always refused, even when offered money.

Living sometimes in sleazy San Francisco hotels (my money was running low) and at other times in sumptuous university residences, was not conducive to dietary control. The best and cheapest meals on the west coast were served in the steakhouses – $3.95 for a thick grilled steak with a big baked potato and salad (all fine for a diabetic), and a huge stein of disastrously sweet American beer.

In the middle of 1971 I returned to Canberra to take up my position at the ANU. I was provided with a three-bedroom house for my companion and me at a very low rent. These were the last days of academic affluence. It was perhaps a mile and half from the house to the university. Nowadays I would walk; then, I used the car. It was some time before the jogging, walking and cycling crazes hit Australia, and in Canberra in particular, we drove everywhere.

I settled into the kind of lifestyle I was to follow, to my very great cost, for the next few years. The work was not taxing and thoroughly enjoyable. There was plenty of time for lunches with wine, drinks after work at the Staff Centre and dinners in restaurants and the homes of our friends. Money was not a problem. My partner and I earned good salaries and we drove and flew frequently to Sydney for weekends to spend time going to parties and restaurants with people equally well off. It was a time of great optimism with the conservative government on its last legs under the ineffectual McMahon, the Australian participation in the Vietnam war clearly winding down and the sexual and social liberation of the sixties unthreatened.

I had not seen an endocrinologist since leaving Melbourne five years before and made no attempt to contact one in Canberra. I can't account for this stupidity unless it was a suspicion that loose living was going to have consequences I did not want to face. Again, I'm looking at myself like a character in a novel, but it might have been so.

I was not totally without medical supervision at this time. I had to have an eyesight test each year to keep my driver's licence, but this was done perfunctorily by a GP. I obtained prescriptions for insulin from the same doctor, but he never subjected me to a full examination or asked questions about my regimen (I followed none, apart from injecting the insulin and avoiding the obviously forbidden foods). At about this time, very belatedly, I became aware that the urine testing strips available were a considerable improvement on the old eye dropper, test tube and tablet method.

The procedure was to dip the strip in a urine sample, but I was certainly not the only diabetic to piss directly onto it for convenience. Whether this affected the result I don't know; urine testing was ineffective anyhow.

Had I only known it, considerable improvements had been made in other areas of treatment and management of diabetes. The glucometer, enabling diabetics to accurately test the blood sugar at any time of the day, was available. It was expensive but I would have been able to afford it. Disposable syringes made the whole injection procedure much less cumbersome, and the glucometer was awakening doctors to the fact that much better control was achieved by multiple injections. Due to my own neglect, I knew nothing of this and continued to follow the outmoded practices of the '50s.

In a sense, I had been brainwashed to rigidly inject the same amount of insulin at the same times each day. I later learned that more mature and aware diabetics, such as Dr Noel McLachlan, my former colleague at Monash, vary their insulin dose according to daily activity and behaviour. Had I done this I might have avoided some of the pain that was in store but, foolishly, I was uninterested in diabetes and treated it as a nuisance rather than as something to manage in my own best interests.

Paradoxically, I slept well, rarely caught colds or flu, and could work all day and play well into the night without apparent ill effect. I was somewhat concerned that I was gaining weight – the result of high calories in the alcohol and reduced physical activity – but again I did not know that the heavier the person, the more insulin is required to keep sugar levels under control. Diabetics should stay thin, and though not fat, I was not thin either. Vascular damage was certainly being done but I was more concerned from a vanity point of view – I disliked the softening of my chin and waist.

So occasionally I played tennis and thought about taking more exercise, even attempting once to scull on Lake Burley Griffin under the guidance of friends who were expert rowers. I was unable to balance the boat, fell in and gave up. I also had a go at squash and disliked it. Mostly, I tried to hold my head at a higher angle and suck my stomach in.

Early in 1972 I went to Papua New Guinea en route to the Solomon Islands to continue work on the labour trade and related topics. There I met Jean Bedford, who I was to live with for the next 11 years and ultimately marry, although not without considerable drama along the way[3].

This time in the Solomons I was taking a little better care of myself and drinking less out of vanity, wanting to present well to Jean. My weight fell to a possibly too light 11 stone (70kg) and I was walking miles every day under a tropic sun. I overdid it. As I now know, the lower the body weight, the less insulin required, but I was injecting the same amount as always.

One day, on San Cristobal, after walking several miles in the heat to reach a point where I could catch a boat, I fell asleep in the shade behind a shed. I slept deeply and my sugar level dropped dramatically, throwing me into the most severe hypo I had experienced in years. I awoke wringing wet, unable to stand and confused to the point of imbecility. There was no-one around but in any case I would have been unable to communicate anything coherent.

I fell asleep again, convinced that I was going to die and desperately sorry that I would never see Jean again. When the body is stressed, as mine certainly was, the liver secretes glucose to enable it to cope. I came out of the sleep just sufficiently alert to claw open my bag and shovel in the few pieces of barley sugar I could find. I had been given a tube of sweetened condensed milk in a mission, which I had not used because its sugar content was so high. Now, I pierced the top with a match and almost sucked it dry. Slowly, my strength came back and with it clarity of mind. I was able to compose myself enough to get down to the wharf and catch the boat.

It had been a near thing. I was lying where no-one could have seen me and if I had not had the barley sugar and sweetened milk I could not have attracted attention. Convulsions and exposure could have done for me.

The subject of diabetes came up early on in my relationship with Jean. Clare Golson, the charming, extroverted wife of Jack Golson, Head of the Archaeology Department at the ANU, had been a nurse. The Golsons were visiting Port Moresby.

'A diabetic?' she said to Jean. 'Nothing but trouble. Don't have any-thing to do with him.'

Happily, Jean ignored the advice. As far as she could see I was a fit, lean, almost-thirty-year-old with no discernible frailties. In those early weeks we spent together I was careful to avoid hypos, using what I called the 'piss strips' to monitor the sugar level and probably keeping it too high too much of the time. I injected in private and minimised the fuss about sterilisation, needles and insulin. I did not tell Jean about the near-disastrous hypo in the Solomons, and reassured her by saying that Clare's perceptions were out of date. I had been diabetic for 15 years and thought it had done me no harm, apart from weakening my eyesight. I was a Doctor of Philosophy, a much-published academic who could drink, dance (after a fashion) and play tennis a bit.

Jean left New Guinea to live with me in Canberra, bringing her three-year-old daughter, Sofya. We spent some time in Melbourne, avoiding the hostility of my former partner. Early one winter morning I left Melbourne to drive to Canberra in a day with a fuel stop at Albury. It was still dark for the first few hours of the drive and I remember having some difficulty in seeing the road. At Kilburn, on the outskirts of the city, it was foggy and I had to make several stops because of the poor visibility. I had driven through fog often enough before without trouble and should have known something was wrong.

I found Sofya a joy and Jean and I were keen to have a child of our own. We struck a snag when a test I had, after months of apparent failure, showed that I had an extremely low sperm count: virtually nil. We were told that this was 'not uncommon' with diabetics and had just reconciled ourselves to having one child only, when Jean almost immediately became pregnant. It transpired that she had washed the bottle into which I had contributed the sample, and this had killed the sperm. My sperm count, in fact, was normal. Our daughter, Miriam, was born in October 1973 and two years later we had another daughter, Ruth.

Canberra winters are severe and I seemed to be less healthy than before. After going rabbit shooting on a particularly bleak day I got a heavy cold; a chest infection with other complications set in soon after. I became very ill, despite Jean's nursing, and sank into something like a coma after taking less insulin than normal and eating less – an ignorant strategy. Jean called a doctor who diagnosed the infection and wrote out a prescription.

'By the way, he's a diabetic,' she said as the doctor was leaving.

That put an entirely different spin on things. The doctor called an emergency ambulance and I was hospitalised in a most dangerous condition: a diabetic with high blood sugar and ketosis poisoning. I responded quickly to insulin and glucose injections as the doctors monitored my blood sugar, the antibiotics in combat with the infections.

Not long after I was released from hospital I encountered two of the doctors who had treated me. I was at the university staff club drinking beer and smoking. They shook their heads and told me how close I had come to dying; it appals me now to record that I took no notice.

In my own defence, I believe these doctors erred in not referring me to an endocrinologist. They were young, probably in training only, and would not have had the authority to insist. Certainly no exhaustive tests were conducted on me. Blood tests and bio-chemical screening would have shown alarming irregularities that could have alerted me, but it's impossible to say. I had ignored many warnings before.

In 1974 I was appointed to a lectureship in History at the University of Melbourne. We bought a house in Fitzroy and settled into an inner city lifestyle which involved me taking Sofya to her preschool on the back of my bike. The area was flat so the going wasn't hard, but the exercise must have helped offset the factors that were potentially disastrous for a diabetic, particularly my ever-increasing alcohol consumption.

We entertained frequently at the Fitzroy house, which had a kind of patio at the back with a grapevine growing all around it. I remember lunches in that pleasant, leafy area... the Lebanese food, with its difficult-to-calculate carbohydrate content, pasta (certainly too much), Chinese dishes, inevitably containing sugar and honey – and drink. Mostly wine and beer, but during one notable session with Jean's old friend Phillip Frazer, who had just flown in from New York, ouzo!

After a year at Melbourne University and another at the Gippsland Institute of Advanced Education, my romance with academic life was over.

Times had changed, annual examinations as the sole means of assessment were out and progressive assessment was in. The old elitist, competitive idea of the university in which I'd thrived was breaking down and I couldn't adjust. I had begun to write book reviews for newspapers and magazines and was getting a kick out of the quick publication. I was also trying my hand at fiction. At the end of 1975 we sold up in Melbourne and moved to Sydney.

Chapter Eleven
GOING BLIND

retinopathy: any disorder of the retina resulting in the impairment of vision. It is usually due to damage to the blood vessels of the retina, occurring (for example) as a complication of diabetes...

Concise Oxford Medical Dictionary

About halfway through 1976, I was pushing Miriam in a stroller through Glebe, when I became aware of spots in front of my eyes. I had noticed something like this a few times before, but it would seem to clear up and I thought nothing of it. Now the spots appeared bigger and mobile and were interfering with my vision. I blinked and rubbed my eyes but this had no effect. I was having trouble focusing and getting a clear image, even of objects quite close to me.

I had always known that long-term diabetes had an effect on the eyesight and had resented the loss of acuity I had suffered early on. But I hadn't calculated on more serious threats to my vision and, alarmed, I telephoned Dr Taft in Melbourne. He must have been surprised to hear from me after so many years, but when I told him of the problem he referred me to Dr Warren Kidson, an endocrinologist in Randwick, urging me to see him as soon as possible.

Dr Kidson, presumably out of respect for Pincus Taft, who was a revered man in the field, gave me an almost immediate appointment. He examined me and was concerned enough to refer me to Dr Paul Beaumont, a Macquarie Street ophthalmologist, again urgently.

I distinctly remember that first appointment in Paul Beaumont's crowded rooms. I arrived on time at 2pm, expecting to be seen almost at once. Instead

I found that, after submitting to some preliminary examinations from a team of highly efficient female technicians, and leaving a urine sample, I had to wait what seemed like an interminable time while elderly, obese diabetics, as well as some younger people and non-diabetics, filed through.

I have always been impatient by nature and the wait went on for so long that I was offended and seriously considered leaving, but eventually I was taken in to see Paul, who conducted a long and detailed examination of my eyes through some elaborate and rather frightening equipment. His conclusion was that I had very severe retinopathy, a condition common among poorly-controlled diabetics. With this disorder, the delicate, peripheral blood vessels to the retina haemorrhage, leaking blood onto it. The eye vessels may also grow haphazardly, become scarred and obscure the vision. Scarred vessels can pull the retina off.

My case was severe and I later learned that the doctors considered removing my pituitary gland, a procedure suited to a kind of retinopathy called 'diffuse capillary retinopathy'. A side-effect of that would have been a decrease in libido, requiring hormone replacement therapy to compensate. Happily, I had few features of this type of the disease: my particular kind of retinopathy responded well to laser treatment and so pituitary removal was not necessary.

A few years earlier I would certainly have gone blind, but the technique of treating retinopathy with an argon laser beam had been introduced to Australia by Associate Professor Fred Hollows, who was Head of the Ophthalmology Department at the University of New South Wales and Prince Henry Hospital in 1972. Paul Beaumont was then the Senior Registrar at the Prince of Wales eye clinic, looking after diabetics. As Paul recalls:

'Fred, with his characteristic ability to delegate, just said, "It's all yours" and allowed me to go full steam ahead, lasering diabetic eyes... The results, of course, were quite dramatic.'

I consider myself very lucky to have been a patient of the man with the greatest experience in Australia at that time at using the argon laser. As I understand it, the laser beam was used to blot up the blood on the retina and to seal off and burn away the leaking and unwanted blood vessels.

Over the next year, I came to know Paul Beaumont's surgery as well as I knew my own living room. I went for treatment twice a week, never getting away in under three hours. At first I resented this until I discovered that Paul began work at 7am and worked at least 12-hour days. The treatment was anything but pleasant. Initially, drops were put into the eyes to dilate the pupil – apparently a necessary preliminary to taking certain measurements. After a time this made reading difficult and the only way I have ever been able to endure waiting is to read.

Furthermore, I could ill afford these great chunks out of my day as I was earning a scrappy living by book reviewing. Usually I had to read a book and sometimes write the review itself in the waiting room. By some lucky chance, I was able to retain enough vision to permit reading and writing long after most people give up. Paul's nurses would see me reading when many other patients were sitting staring blindly about, and shake their heads.

The laser treatment came in two forms – light and heavy. In the former, the beam touched less sensitive parts of the retina and the procedure was not supposed to be painful. It was though – always. A contact lens attached to a device like a jeweller's glass was inserted and I had to place my chin on a rest and keep perfectly still while the beam was directed into my eye. A treatment lasted for several minutes and was always uncomfortable and stressful, despite Paul's soothing manner. Sometimes it hurt almost as much as having a nerve touched by a dentist's drill.

Having heavy laser necessitated getting a local anaesthetic administered to the bunch of nerves under the eye. The needle coming over and down looked to be three inches, and as the eyes are possibly the most vulnerable organs in the body (apart from the genitals) this invasion was hard to endure. The injection hurt, and while the procedure that followed was not painful, several pain killers had to be administered at the end of it.

A gauze patch over the eye had to remain in place for several hours and rest was advised. Many, many times I stumbled my way to the George Street bus stop, squinting with one eye to read the destination, and staggered back to Wigram Road to collapse and sleep until the throbbing in my eye woke me. Stress raised the metabolic rate and I sometimes neglected to eat enough after a treatment. As a result I would wake from the sleep sweating freely, then slip into a hypo.

Once, I described all this to a friend, who summed it up accurately: 'That's not for squibs'.

Indeed it wasn't. Women frequently wept in the surgery and I never saw anyone who was totally relaxed about the treatment. Paul Beaumont's manner, however, inspired confidence and he was as compassionate and considerate as the technique permitted. As a reader and writer, my vision was of crucial importance, and I never once questioned whether the pain and trauma were worthwhile. Many of the episodes, such as the biopsy, haunt me still. In the biopsy, a section of my arm was frozen, and a piece of tissue about the size of a pea was sliced out. The angiogram was worse. A dye would be injected into the vein to permit study of the flow of blood in the eye. When the dye kicked in I felt intensely nauseous, yet had to remain dead still.

I was frequently incapacitated after laser treatment, returning home shaken and in pain. I had several serious hypos because I found it difficult to eat in this condition.

Paul Beaumont expressed cautious optimism about the effects of the treatment. Although the retinopathy was very severe and the damage extensive, it was in my favour that I was comparatively young and otherwise healthy. I made some efforts to get the diabetes under better control at this time, testing the urine regularly, keeping to the diet and taking more exercise, mostly walking around Glebe and Annandale pushing the stroller. (I walked miles in this way and acquired an intimate knowledge of the streetscape of the area, which I used in the Cliff Hardy novels).

At Paul's insistence, because of its deleterious effects on the blood, I stopped smoking, I had no difficulty doing so, but did not, however, stop drinking, often consuming most of a flagon of wine in a day. I had never smoked when I wrote, but I always drank, and the more I wrote the more I drank.

I was never a binge drinker, just a steady imbiber from early in the morning until late at night. I drank every day. I did not suffer from hangovers, no matter how much cheap wine I drank. It was not uncommon for me to drink wine with my breakfast toast and scrambled eggs (as I heard Mick Jagger did), and I was often at the Harold Park Hotel for a beer shortly after it opened.

I had become heavily dependent on alcohol in connection with writing, socialising and, especially, sex.

After Ruth was born we moved to a bigger house in Glebe. We did the move over a number of days, making innumerable trips with boxes and small items between the two addresses. I worked hard, loading and unloading on a particularly hot day, and obviously did not eat enough. Somewhere along Glebe Point Road I entered the confused twilight zone of the serious hypo and lost all sense of who I was and what I was doing. It was very lucky for me (and other road users) that I became aware of what was happening and managed to stop the car somewhere near the water and consume the plastic-wrapped sugar cubes I at least had the sense to carry with me.

Slowly coming out of the hypo, while still retaining some of its mind-bending qualities, I realised that I had practically been hallucinating like an LSD tripper, vividly imagining streets, intersections and other features that did not exist. Apparently, I had negotiated the real carriageways, but it must have been a near thing. I sat in the hot little car while the sweat ran off me and slowly dried, and reflected that I frequently had all three children with me when driving. I resolved never to drive a car when there was any possibility of my sugar level dropping: one of the few responsible commitments I made and stuck to at that time.

We hired the Glebe identity Tom Laming to do the removal. Tom was the proprietor of The Dealatorium, a large secondhand shop, and also ran the Golden Gloves gymnasium in Arundel Street. He had been a main event boxer in his youth, a light-heavyweight who had twice fought, and lost to, the great Dave Sands. A plaque in the rockery at the top of Glebe Point Road, commemorating Dave Sands, was paid for by Tom Laming.

By this time, however, Tom, a late-life-onset diabetic, was obese. On that hot day in December he drank an entire two-litre bottle of Coca Cola. I shuddered at the thought of what his blood sugar might be.

Chapter Twelve

MEETING FRED HOLLOWS

'If you don't get off the piss and get fit, you'll be blind in five years and dead in 10.'

Fred Hollows, 1978

The turning point in my diabetic life came when I met Fred Hollows. Towards the end of 1978, Jean and I attended a birthday party for Pat Fiske, an American-born film-maker whose documentary on the Builders Labourers Federation was to win many awards. (She went on to make an outstanding film about Hollows.) The party was held in his home, Farnham House.

I had wanted to meet Hollows for some time because of his pioneering role in introducing laser treatment to Australia, and also because I admired the work he'd done in the trachoma program in Aboriginal communities, particularly his defiance of the detestable Bjelke-Petersen. By this time the laser treatments were almost completed and my vision was saved. I had stopped smoking and cut down my drinking, but I was overweight and not taking regular systematic exercise.

Pat introduced me to Fred, a stocky, hardbodied man with a shock of thick grey hair. She said something about diabetes, the laser and Paul Beaumont. He looked at me over the tops of his half-glasses, took the curved pipe out of his mouth, and prodded me hard in my soft belly with his fist.

'What's this gut you've got on you? You've had all this expensive treatment and you're just fucking throwing it away. Diabetics should be thin! If you don't get off the piss and get fit you'll be blind in five years and dead in 10.'

He then asked me what my latest glycosylated haemoglobin reading was, but I didn't know what he was talking about. He turned away in disgust.

I was profoundly shocked. I hadn't been so rudely and abruptly addressed since becoming an adult, and my first reaction was anger and resentment. Who was this little pipe-puffing runt to talk to me like that about fitness and drinking? He probably wasn't stone cold sober himself.

Nevertheless, his words struck home. 'Blind' and 'dead' have a ring to them that can cut through laziness and complacency. Not many days later I got out an old pair of tennis shoes, pulled on shorts and a T-shirt, and set off to run the 200 metres to the Jubilee Park oval and do a few laps. I was astonished to find that I couldn't complete the 200. I conked out, completely puffed, well short of the oval.

Humiliated yet challenged, I felt that at 36 I ought to be able to run a kilometre or two, despite never having been much of a distance runner. I persisted that morning, interspersing jogging with walking, until I had completed about one-and-a-half kilometres.

I went out again the next morning, and the next. I bought a pair of Adidas running shoes and within a couple of weeks was able to jog quietly to the oval and complete four laps. I built it up to 10 and then experienced an agonising pain in my ankles. Hooked on jogging by this time and in despair at having to stop, I hobbled along to the doctor in the Fairfax building, where I was working part-time as Literary Editor of *The National Times*. I was asked where I was running.

'Around a football ground.'

'Good', said the doctor. 'Is it cambered?'

I reflected.

'I guess so, slightly.'

'No problem. You've got tendonitis from running too far, too early. Rest it for a while and then run one lap around one way, and the next the other. You'll be all right.'

I did exactly that and soon was running almost five kilometres every morning – not fast, but without stopping. By now we had a dog, a splendid border collie-cross, and Jim was my companion on these early morning runs. He'd lope along beside me to the oval, complete a few laps, and then run off to chase birds or sit under a tree and watch as I completed my sweaty circuits. He was a magnificent dog – handsome, obedient, playful – and the children adored him. The big block at our new house gave him space to play and dig and do everything dogs do, and he became a favourite of the local shopkeepers, particularly the gay proprietor of a mixed business, who gave him treats.

I bought the *Complete Book of Running* and was inspired by Jim Fixx's account of how he had turned his life around. In a magazine I saw a photo of the old Fixx, flabby and tired-looking, and was astonished at the transformation. Running Jim looked years younger and much happier. I cut down drastically on my drinking and the weight fell away. I ran every day and began to complete the distance in a shorter time, so I ran further.

I had completely caught the running bug: the shoes, the singlet, the shorts, the liniment, the lot. I took my gear to work and ran around Wentworth Park in my lunch break. I abandoned the habit I had picked up from John Morgan and followed ever since in Melbourne, Gippsland and Sydney – that of taking a small tomato sauce bottle full of red wine to drink with my lunch.

If I had gone about it in the right way, this radical change in my lifestyle should have produced nothing but good results – better diabetic control, better health generally, and a considerable saving of money. Trying to limit myself to two or three glasses of wine per day, I had reduced my daily intake of calories by several hundred. If I had consulted Warren Kidson before embarking on the jogging life, he would no doubt have warned me to reduce my insulin to compensate for the lost weight, to eat more to balance the increased activity, and perhaps to lower the insulin dose still further on those mornings when I was running.

I did not consult him and made none of these adjustments, still locked into taking the same amount of insulin each day and eating my six-portion meals with one portion in between. Still worse, I was proud of the lost weight and reluctant to eat more than was necessary to function.

I was utterly ignorant of the mechanics of diabetic control, despite having been a sufferer for 20 years. The result was that I entered a phase, lasting almost a year, of cataclysmic hypos, more serious than I had ever experienced before, which caused great distress to those around me and inflicted grievous damage on my relationship with Jean.

The first of the major hypos happened one morning after running, while taking Ruth to her creche in Forest Lodge and Miriam to her preschool in

Jubilee Park. After shopping and walking home, my blood sugar dropped so quickly and severely that I became too confused to take glucose. I wandered the streets and only arrived home by accident. Somehow I found my way into the house, only to doubt that it *was* my house – nothing seemed familiar.

A most peculiar notion had entered my head. I realised that I was having a hypo but, since I couldn't account for it, decided I must be miraculously cured of diabetes. In some way the pancreas was secreting insulin after 20 years of not doing so, and this plus the injected insulin had thrown me into the hypo.

I was briefly wondrously happy with this explanation and lay down on the bed to enjoy it. The delusion soon passed and I managed to get some barley sugar from my pocket, take it and recover sufficient sense to get to the kitchen for more sugar and food. The bed linen and parts of the mattress were soaked with sweat, and I was a shaky ruin. This was one of the times I attempted (not always successfully) to conceal the hypo from Jean by washing and drying the linen and covering the damp patches on the mattress.

I have several times experienced great joy when in the hypoglycaemic state. I can understand everything in the universe and grasp the real meaning and harmony that governs all things. Fasting and other mortifications, as practised by religious charismatics, result in a lowering of the blood sugar. I conclude that their visions and visitations are delusions, caused by an alteration in the body chemistry.

Once I slipped into hypo when working at the newspaper. It was lunchtime and I had eaten, but evidently not enough. My weight was down, my insulin dose was constant and I had run hard in the morning. There were only a few people in the office as the sweat began to drip from my head onto the desk. I crashed to the ground, upsetting my chair and wrenching my arm as I fell. Luckily, Adele Horin was one of the people there. At that time she was living with Robert Pullan, journalist and anticensorship agitator, who is about my age and has been diabetic for about as long. Adele knew that a can of Coke, if taken in time, could raise the blood sugar quickly. That's what happened. Again, I did not tell Jean about this and swore Adele and the others to secrecy.

I made the same request of the poet Geoff Page, whom I took to lunch on the paper's expense account. The idea was to put a poet on a retainer to select poems to be published in the book pages. I had read no poetry for years and considered myself unqualified, but I liked Page's poetry and would trust his judgment. Again, after a morning run and a busy time at the paper, my sugar level dropped so that I was soon sweating as if in a sauna, and making no sense at all. As we were in a restaurant, sugar was on the table and I spooned enough in to bring myself out of the hypo.

I explain things to Page, who said that his first thought was that I was a junkie attempting to get off heroin by going cold turkey.

I couldn't conceal this state of affairs for very long, especially after experiencing several very severe hypos after falling asleep at night. On these occasions Jean was unable to get me to take sugar and was forced to call an ambulance and enlist the aid of the paramedics.

These incidents naturally caused Jean great distress. She couldn't trust me when the children were in my sole care, as they frequently were, and when she flew to Melbourne after her mother suffered a series of strokes and apparently did not have long to live, she had to arrange for friends to stay with me and the girls. But she did not feel she could impose too long on the friends and flew back – on a night when the most severe of these hypos hit.

Usually, the paramedics were able to inject glucose and bring me around but this time, when I had terrified Jean by shouting and throwing myself violently around the room, bouncing off and bloodying the walls, she had to take the children next door. I fought the ambulance men like a berserker, but remember nothing of this. A second team had to be called to overpower me and I emerged from this episode with a broken collarbone and a torn arm, from thrashing about and resisting the glucose needle.

Through literary agent Tim Curnow came the offer of two long articles on the search Ruth Park and her late husband D'arcy Niland had conducted in America for people there who had known Les Darcy. I was the obvious person to vet the articles and to select photographs from the large collection Ruth had at her house in Palm Beach. It was a hot day when I travelled up there by bus and walked a fair distance to the house.

She was charming and amusing and we got down to work on the selection. That is almost all I remember of the meeting.

Later, when I woke up in the casualty ward at Royal Prince Alfred, I had a dim recollection of a taxi. Apparently, after we had picked the photos and made arrangements to have them copied, I had become confused and Ruth had called for a taxi to take me to the bus stop. In the taxi, just before the hypo hit with full force, I asked the driver to take me to Glebe. On the way I sweated and raved and he took me to the nearest hospital to home – again, RPA. He also took 20 dollars from my pocket for his fare.

The doctors in Casualty expressed great concern at my condition. It had taken a massive injection of glucose to bring me around and they wanted to know why I hadn't taken the glucose tablets I was carrying, and why I had nothing on me to indicate I was a diabetic. The answer to the first question was that these hypos were so sudden and severe that I became too confused too quickly to act rationally. The answer to the second was bravado and irresponsibility.

Chapter Thirteen
GETTING BETTER

'You came very close to the tin cup and the white cane.'

Dr Warren Kidson, 1979

Alarmed by my condition, the doctors called in Dr John Burgess, a distinguished endocrinologist who had rooms in the hospital's medical centre. Not surprisingly, I have little recollection of our first meeting. John has since told me that the hypo was so severe that initially I was disoriented and would have had difficulty remembering events over the previous 24 hours, and for some time later. He suggested it might be more convenient for me to see him than Warren Kidson, given that I lived so close in Glebe.

This was insightful of him. The truth was that I was not keeping in as regular contact with Dr Kidson as I should have done. The doctors sorted the matter out between them and I became John's patient.

I found him sympathetic but not without severity. I told him of my drinking habits, which still were not always under control, and of my history of retinopathy, hypos and the recently adopted fitness fetish. He recommended that I change my regimen to one involving three injections per day: Actrapid, the insulin that lowered blood sugar quickly, before breakfast and lunch; this plus Monotard, a slower acting insulin, before the evening meal.

The object was to approximate more closely the way the body naturally produces insulin to cope with the intake of food. Of course, the amount of activity remained a variable, but it was far safer to run in the morning after a smaller dose of insulin than it had been previously after the dose designed to last most of the whole day. I have continued to consult with John Burgess or an endocrinologist once a year and to have extensive blood tests to monitor my condition.

Twenty years after the initial diagnosis, I began to adopt a responsible attitude towards the disease.

This change spelled an end to the incapacitating, hospitalising hypos, but out of vanity, pride in my new fitness and sheer stubbornness, I continued to run too much and too far and eat too little. I was testing more frequently and trying to achieve a better balance, but I was still ignorant of many of the elements of control.

The 'piss strips', improperly used, yielded unreliable results and I frequently miscalculated. I still had severe hypos, so Jean's fears were not allayed, and after the many deceptions I had practised (including concealing ambulance and hospital bills from her), she was understandably distrustful of me.

Although John Burgess inspired confidence, this was not true of all his colleagues. Some time after coming under Dr Burgess' care I went into hospital to have a vasectomy. I had the operation under a general anaesthetic and, despite having advised the doctors about my diabetes, I came around to find that I was receiving a glucose solution through a drip. I pulled the needle out and tested my urine, only to find that the sugar level was sky-high. I spent hours then walking up and down the corridor in a rage, insisting that I needed the activity to reduce the blood sugar. I had been told that the aftermath of the operation was like a 'kick in the nuts', but I suffered no such discomfort. Perhaps I was too angry to notice.

My reaction to this medical foul-up was a positive sign. I had begun to care passionately about good control and I resented every urine test that was above the accepted range. I was seeing diabetes as a central fact in my life and the management of it as essential to my well-being and happiness, and my effectiveness as a parent.

Jean and I moved to Coledale on the south coast and I continued with my fitness program, running along the coast road fringing the beach, swimming and running back. In fact I became obsessed with it and swam all year round, whatever the weather. I managed to cut down on my drinking and, with a lot of grass to mow, wood to chop, and some water-carrying for Sofya's horse,

I became fitter than I'd ever been. The diabetic control improved markedly and when I reported to Paul Beaumont on the anniversary of the end of my laser treatment he pronounced the retinopathy 'quiet' and congratulated me.

After 20 years as a diabetic I had finally earned some praise for my discipline. It meant a great deal to me and it was confirmed by the blood tests which were to become an annual event under Dr Burgess' direction. For probably the first time in 15 years I was in a fairly sound biochemical condition. My eyesight was irreparably damaged: I had lost most of my peripheral vision and the capacity to adapt quickly to changes in the degree of light. But it was functional and I had sufficient acuity to continue to hold a driver's licence. Other damage and disturbances would emerge as years went by, but I had pulled out of the spiral that would have left me blind and incapacitated. As Dr Kidson said, in a phrase that has remained with me ever since: 'You came very close to the tin cup and the white cane.'

Chapter Fourteen
GOING STRAIGHT

Lush is a testimony to the value of insulin. After a lifetime of receiving the hormone her body could not provide she was more active than most women her age. She was trim, attractive and wore fashionable clothes with taste and style.

> — obituary of Mrs Phyllis Lush, 1916-98,
> *The Australian,* 6 July, 1998.

If meeting Fred Hollows provided the psychological and emotional stimulus for me to take responsibility for my diabetes, technical improvements in the 1970s and '80s helped the process along. I can't remember exactly when I switched from the glass and metal hypodermic (with all the attendant maintenance and storage hassles) to disposable syringes, but it was liberating to do so. Somehow, the light, cheap throwaway syringes made the whole process seem less of a nuisance.

It certainly made it easier to inject while visiting or eating out. I suspect most diabetics get a few more injections out of each syringe than just one, but I never use them so that they became blunt. Provided very cheaply by a government-backed scheme, they offer no incentive to be over-economical.

As mentioned before, the great breakthrough in daily management came with the glucometer. Compared to the units available today, only half the size of a cigarette packet, my first glucometer was a clumsy affair. Bought in the early 1980s, it cost $500, which was a stretch for me at the time. It was easy to use and accurate, however, and allowed much greater flexibility in balancing the key elements of control – diet, insulin and exercise. As it happened, that glucometer, perhaps resembling an electric shaver or some such useful item when zipped into its carry bag, was stolen.

By this time I was a fairly well-known writer and I managed to get an item on my loss printed in 'Column 8' of *the Sydney Morning Herald,* but there was no response. I had to take out a loan to buy another one because there was no way I was going to be without it. Nowadays, the glucometers cost less than $100 and it's possible to have one at home and one at work or one for travelling. Like insulin and the syringes, the testing strips are subsidised and comparatively cheap. I sometimes test four or five times a day when I feel the need to know exactly how the blood sugar level is moving.

While I haven't read a great deal about the disease, I did finally read *The Diabetic Life,* and reviewed a recent excellent book: *Understanding Diabetes: Managing Your Life with Diabetes,* for a Brisbane newspaper.[4] I watch the press for reports on research into the disease and try to stay abreast through such programs as the ABC's *Health Report.* I'm not a 'joiner' so I've never been active in the superb work done by Diabetes Australia, but I did give the guest address at a recent conference held by the organisation in Sydney. I was also delighted, when asked by Dr Kidson, to contribute a story to the magazine *Conquest,* to knock out a Cliff Hardy yarn involving a young diabetic. I didn't do much in the way of research, but as a way of giving thanks for my lucky escape, I give a regular donation to the New South Wales Guide Dogs Association appeal.

Diabetes is on the increase and it's estimated that there are as many undiagnosed diabetics in the community as those who are being treated. These people are in danger of the most severe consequences – blindness, impotence, loss of limbs – and I am happy to stress these dangers when asked to make statements to this effect. In 1998 I gave a talk at the Redlands Community Hospital to a group of diabetic patients, mostly, but not all, Type-2 sufferers. This group met regularly with nurses, doctors and dieticians, as well as occasional blowins like me, and I was impressed by their knowledge and the responsible way they went about insuring their lives and their usefulness because that's what the proper management of diabetes comes down to. I also liked their senses of humour – they laughed at my jokes.

My research into the disease included noting prominent people who suffered from it: HG Wells, Ernest Hemingway and Peter Lalor, the hero of the Eureka Stockade, among many others. I wrote an article for *The National*

Times in which I interviewed some diabetics and got their stories, among them the late Norm Gallagher, former strongman of the Builder's Labourers Federation, and the remarkable Mrs Phyllis Lush.

Mrs Lush developed diabetes in 1921 at the age of five and her father secured an early batch of insulin from Canada from the laboratory of Drs Banting and Best, who'd made the discovery. The insulin arrived wrapped in cotton wool, in the care of the purser of a P&O liner. When she received her first injection she weighed less than 10 kilograms and was close to death. An energetic and disciplined person, Mr Lush later married a doctor and lived for 76 years, enjoying good health until near the end. *The Guinness Book of Records* credits her as the longest known surviving insulin-dependent diabetic. Her story should be made known to all diabetics for its inspirational value.

Like all writers, I've drawn on my personal experience in producing my books. The mother of my fictional detective, Cliff Hardy, I've drawn as a poorly controlled diabetic creating unwanted drama in young Cliff's life. Diabetes figures in the first of the Hardy novels, *The Dying Trade*, but most prominently in *Cross Off,* in which a ruthless hit man, a diabetic, has a hypo at a most inconvenient time.

> Another shot almost had him. He was drenched in sweat and his fingers slipped on the pistol grip. He ducked down and suddenly felt his vision blur and his strength ebb. He rubbed his hands across his eyes. He couldn't focus... He'd forgotten to eat midmorning and all the activity and excitement had sent his blood sugar plummeting. He felt in his pocket for barley sugar but he had none. Must have dropped it. In a few minutes he'd be as weak as a kitten. He needed sugar fast.

I've been there. I knew how to write that scene.

Chapter Fifteen

LIFE WITH DIABETES WASN'T MEANT TO BE EASY

'Diabetes is an immune system disorder and immune system disorders tend to cluster.'

Dr Paul Beaumont, October 1999

The consequences of poorly controlled diabetes are disastrous. In my case, even once I'd committed myself to achieving and maintaining good control, things continued to go wrong. Diabetics commonly develop cataracts which, in days gone by, meant they suffered restricted vision and had to wear thick-lensed glasses.

Cataracts developed in both my eyes and required treatment by the mid-1980s. Luckily for me, again, the technology had improved: the implanting of intra-ocular lenses, replacing the lens that has become opaque, could restore a patient's normal vision. The IOLs, implanted in a quick operation under local anaesthetic, have given me the vision I presently enjoy. It's far from perfect, but I can drive, watch films and hit a golf ball – sometimes. I don't wear glasses to read.

The work begun by Fred Hollows and continued by the Fred Hollows Foundation, has brought the benefits of this technology to Eritrea, Nepal and Vietnam. Previously, cataract sufferers in Third World countries could not afford the lenses and there were no surgeons competent at the operation. Hollows pioneered the teaching of the technique to Third World doctors and the Foundation's lens factories in Eritrea and Vietnam are producing the lenses at an affordable price.

Thirteen years after our first meeting, when he had treated me with the contempt I'd deserved, I met Fred Hollows again. I was commissioned to help him write his autobiography. I got the job because I had a reputation for writing quickly and time appeared to be short as Fred was suffering from advanced cancer. This time we got on well and work on the book progressed rapidly. We finished it within the time Fred had been expected to live and in fact he survived for a further 18 months, enabling him to promote the book. This promotion – and Fred's involvement in several controversies at the end of his life – helped it to become a best-seller. At last count it had sold more than 100,000 copies, most of the proceeds going to the Foundation.

I had a series of blood tests while I was working on the book and couldn't wait to tell Fred my glycosylated haemoglobin readings – a very good, 6.1 result.

I reminded him of what he'd said at our first meeting and he clapped me on the shoulder. 'Good boy,' he growled. It's a moment I treasure.

As things stand I'm routinely congratulated by my endocrinologist and oph-thalmologist on my good health. Paul Beaumont – who sees no reason why I shouldn't retain my present vision for the rest of my life – chilled me when he told me some years ago that the prognosis for a diabetic presenting with retinopathy as severe as mine had been in 1977, was 'the same as for someone with stomach cancer – six months'. This is because most such patients would have been much older than I was, obese and unable or unwilling to change their habits.

I do have various biochemical disturbances to contend with – low thyroid activity and a raised prolactin level among them. These are con-trolled by medication. More recently I have been diagnosed as having a gluten intolerance, a common occurrence among diabetics. It is an immune-system-related condition, which diabetes is coming to be seen as, and such conditions tend to occur in clusters. Gluten intolerance, or coeliac disease, if untreated, inhibits the body's ability to absorb certain vitamins and minerals and can increase the risk of cancer and osteoporo-sis. Happily, the treatment is simple: the adoption of a gluten-free diet. These days gluten-free breads, biscuits, cereals and pastas are readily available, so the inconvenience is minimal – although the extra expense is annoying.

Like most long-term diabetics I've suffered a certain degree of vascular damage which has reduced my ability to achieve and maintain an erection. A recent survey showed that only a tiny proportion of Australian men experiencing difficulties with potency seek medical advice. This is the height of ignorance and stupidity. Simple and completely effective therapy is available to solve this problem.

CONCLUSION

In one of the best book launch speeches I've ever heard, Frank Moorhouse advanced the idea that published writers should be compelled to contribute a biopsy, a tissue sample, for preservation in the National Library. Critics of the future, he asserted, might learn more about the mainsprings of their creativity from this than from minute study of their works.

Moorhouse was joking of course, but in fact there has recently been a considerable interest in the medical condition of writers. William B Ober's brilliant book, *Boswell's Clap and Other Essays: Medical Analyses of Literary Men's Afflictions*,[5] is an example. Apart from Boswell's venereal disease, Ober discusses Swinburne's masochism, the madness of certain eighteenth century poets and Rochester's premature ejaculation, amusingly and with some critical effect. Tom Dadis' *The Thirsty Muse*,[6] is a revealing study of the alcoholism of Fitzgerald, Flemingway, O'Neill and other American writers.

Mostly, the writers themselves have been too busy going about their creative work to discuss their medical conditions, but John O'Hara wrote about his addiction to cigarettes, Gore Vidal has mentioned his drinking and William Styron has written penetratingly about his life-and-death struggle with depressions.[7] While not keen to place myself among these giants, it might be of some interest for me to have contributed this account of the disease that has been central to my existence. I have indicated the overt use of it I've made in my writing, but whether it has had more deep-seated effects, I cannot say.

If forced to attempt to analyse the psychological effects of the disease on my behaviour, I arrive at an uncomfortable conclusion: I was ashamed of being a diabetic, as if it betrayed some moral as well as physical weakness. This, perhaps more than anything else, led me sadly astray.

I conclude this account with one piece of advice, particularly aimed at the carers of young diabetics: convince the kid that despite all the advances in knowledge and treatment, the cause of *diabetes mellitus* is still a mystery, like life itself, and that having the bloody disease is a nuisance and a challenge, but nothing to be ashamed of.

REFERENCES

[1] Such as *Understanding Diabetes: Managing your life with diabetes,* The Diabetes Centre, St Vincent's Hospital, Sydney: Simon & Schuster, 1997.

[2] As an example, medical opinion about the complications associated with diabetes was not exactly optimistic. The *Methuen Concise Encyclopaedia of Science and Technology,* published in 1978, states: 'eye complications should be recognised early, especially in juvenile onset cases, as early intervention may prevent or delay blindness.' p 166

[3] Jean and I were both married when we met in 1972. We lived together for 11 years without marrying and then separated. By then we were both divorced. Jean married again and I entered a relationship with another woman. Jean's husband died and my relationship ended. We got back together again in 1990 and married in 1991.

[4] *Sunday Mail Magazine*, 16 November 1997

[5] London: Alison & Busby, 1988

[6] New York, 1989

[7] *Darkness Visible,* New York, 1990

AFTERWORD

I have been asked to add a few words about this book, concerning the interface between the social and scientific aspects of diabetes, and the advances in science and technology which have occurred since Peter Corris was diagnosed as a diabetic 42 years ago. Having had Type-1 (insulin dependent) diabetes myself for 40 years, since I was a medical student, I can easily identify with the problems Peter has faced, such as coping with hypoglycaemia during university exams, sport, loss of self-confidence, and having doubts about the ability to succeed in my chosen profession. Like Peter, I have also tried to conceal hypoglycaemia due to embarrassment and, like Peter, have found that one's saviour from severe hypoglycaemia is usually a woman (men usually think you are drunk, or are too embarrassed to say anything!).

Improvements in our understanding of diabetes, and in technology, have made it a lot easier to live with in recent years. The greatest single advance in patient management was the introduction of home blood glucose monitoring in 1978, arguably the most significant step forward since the discovery of insulin in 1921. Prior to this, diabetics relied on urine glucose tests which were at best unhelpful, and often frankly misleading. The early glucometers were bulky desktop devices, but modern monitors are small enough to be carried in a coat pocket or small handbag, and are more accurate and reliable. Attempts are being made to develop a continuous blood glucose monitoring device which can be worn like a wrist watch (and this would be of immense benefit) but the models currently available are too inaccurate and too expensive to operate for most patients.

The glycosylated haemoglobin (HBA1c) assay, also introduced in the late 1970s, gives valuable and reliable information about overall blood glucose control over the preceding two to three months. It is particularly useful in identifying patients who falsify their blood glucose record in an effort to mislead their parents and doctors into believing they are compliant with treatment strategies.

It has been possible to measure plasma insulin levels by radioimmunoassay since the 1960s; understanding the fluctuations which occur in insulin levels during the day has led to the development of insulin regimens which more closely mimic the insulin levels in the non-diabetic, such as the basal-bolus regimen of four injections per day – these have made it much easier to achieve satisfactory diabetic control. Rapid acting insulin analogues are now available, eg. LisPro (Humalog) and Insulin Aspart (NovoRapid), which provide better control of blood glucose after meals than conventional insulins; long-acting insulin analogues are currently in clinical trial.

Injector pens were introduced in 1985 to cope with the basal-bolus insulin regimen, and have largely replaced syringes except where long acting insulins or mixtures are required. Continuous insulin infusion devices for home use were first described more than 20 years ago, but their usefulness is limited by considerations of cost and inconvenience.

We can now measure circulating antibodies in children of insulin dependent diabetics, and predict with considerable accuracy which children are at risk of developing diabetes. Strategies to delay or prevent overt diabetes from developing are being trialed. In 2000 the 'cure' is still elusive, but advances in DNA technology should soon lead to the production of artificial Beta cells which can be implanted, and which will release insulin when the blood glucose rises above normal. We live in exciting times.

Peter Corns' account of the life and experiences of an insulin-dependent diabetic is fascinating and easy to read. His description of the 'denial' of diabetes and the risk of complications ('it won't happen to me') will be immensely valuable to young people or those with newly diagnosed diabetes who are having difficulty coping with injections, fingerpricks and the need for a regulated lifestyle. Parents of young diabetics will also learn a lot about the tortured thought processes of their children as they struggle to come to terms with their diabetes – and make no mistake, it *is* a struggle!

Diabetes nurse educators are generally much better than doctors at teaching patients how to live with diabetes, and if there is any deficiency in this book, it is that the importance of diabetes educators is not given enough prominence.

One final comment: There is a distressing tendency to use political correctness (aka political idiocy) and refer to the diabetic as a Person with Diabetes or PWD. Personally I believe the use of the term PWD is one form of denial of diabetes, and am delighted that the straight talking and disarmingly honest Peter Corris calls himself a diabetic. Long may he flourish!

Dr Alan E Stocks A.M.
MB., BS(London) MRCS.,
LRCP., MRACP., FRACP., FRCP.

Emeritus Consultant Physician, Princess Alexandra
Hospital, Brisbane
Clinical Associate Professor, University of Queensland

President, Australian Diabetes Society 1980-82
Patron, Diabetic Association of Qld 1972-87
Governor, Kellion Diabetes Foundation

May, 2000

GLOSSARY

Beta cells:	the insulin producing cells of the pancreas
Cardiovascular:	pertaining to the heart and blood vessels
Cataract:	an opacity in the lens of the eye
Coma:	loss of consciousness from any cause. In diabetes from very high or very low blood glucose levels
Diabetes:	disease in which the body cannot produce insulin or use insulin properly. Characterised by high blood glucose levels
Erectile dysfunction:	See Impotence
Glucometer:	blood glucose monitoring unit
Glucose:	the form of sugar found in the human body
Glycosylated haemoglobin reading:	test that gives accurate reading of overall blood glucose control over last 2-3 months
Haemoglobin:	the red coloured iron protein that carries oxygen in red cells
Hyperglycaemia:	blood glucose higher than normal
Hypoglycaemia:	blood glucose level lower than normal
Impotence:	the inability in males to start, sustain or complete the act of sexual intercourse

Insulin:	a hormone produced by the pancreas that lowers blood glucose
Insulin Dependent Diabetes:	See Type-1 diabetes
Juvenile Onset Diabetes:	See Type-1 diabetes
Ketones:	chemical substances from the breakdown of fat which can be dangerous in large amounts
Maturity (late) Onset Diabetes:	See Type-2 diabetes
Non-Insulin Dependent Diabetes:	See Type-2 diabetes
Pancreas:	a gland lying towards the back of the abdomen half-way between the navel and line joining the nipples
Plasma:	the liquid portion of blood
Type-1 Diabetes:	where little or no insulin is made, usually occurring under the age of 30 and requiring insulin injections for life. Also known as insulin dependent and juvenile onset diabetes
Type-2 Diabetes	Insulin is present but doesn't work adequately. Usually occurs over the age of 30 and is controlled by diet and medication or diet and insulin. Also known as non-insulin dependent and maturity onset diabetes.

RESOURCES LIST - DIABETES AUSTRALIA

Australian Capital Territory

Diabetes Australia – ACT
The Grant Cameron
Community Centre
Mulley Street
HOLDER ACT 2611

PO Box 3727
WESTON CREEK ACT
2611

Ph: 02 6288 9830
Fax: 02 6288 9874

New South Wales

Diabetes Australia – NSW
26 Arundel Street
GLEBE NSW 2037

GPO Box 9824
SYDNEY NSW 2001

Ph: 08 8234 1977
Fax: 08 8234 2013
Email:
dasa@da-sa.com.au

South Australia

Diabetes Australia – SA
Unit 4, 159 Burbridge Road
HILTON SA 5033

GPO Box 1930
ADELAIDE SA 5001

Ph: 03 9654 8777
Fax: 03 9650 1917
Email: dav@peg.apc.org

Western Australia

Diabetes Australia –WA
48 Wickham Street
PERTH WA 6004

Ph: 08 9325 7699
Fax: 08 9221 1183

Victoria

Diabetes Australia – VIC
3rd Floor, 100 Collins Street
(PO Box 9824)
MELBOURNE VIC 3000

Queensland

Diabetes Australia – QLD
Cnr Ernest & Merivale
Street
SOUTH BRISBANE QLD
4101

PO Box 3814
SOUTH BRISBANE MAC
QLD 4101

Ph: 07 3239 5666
Fax: 07 3846 4642
Email: ea@daq.org.au

Tasmania

Diabetes Australia – TAS
57E Brisbane Street
HOBART TAS 7000

Ph: 03 6234 5223
Fax: 02 6234 5828
Email:
DATAS@bigpond.com.au

Northern Territory

Diabetes Australia – NT
2 Tiwi Place
TIWI NT 0810

GPO Box 40113
CASUARINA NT 0811

Ph: 08 8297 8488/
08 8927 8482
Fax: 08 8927 8515